Members of the Working Party on Preventive Medicine

Dame Margaret E. H. Turner-Warwick DBE DM PRCP (*President*)

H. P. Lambert MD FRCP FRCPath FFPHM (*Chairman*)

Jocelyn O. P. Chamberlain FRCP FFPHM (*Honorary Secretary*)

J. G. Avery MD FFPHM

D. Cohen BCom MPhil

G. H. Fowler OBE FRCGP

A. M. Dawson MD FRCP

J. Grimley Evans MD FRCP FFPHM

A. P. Haines MD MRCP(UK) MFPHM MRCGP

W. W. Holland MD FRCP FRCGP PFPHM

D. G. Julian MD FRCP

E. B. Macdonald MRCP(UK) FFOM

N. D. Noah FRCP FFPHM

Catherine S. Peckham MD FRCP FRCPath FFPHM

B. W. Taylor PhD FRCP

Observer

J. M. Graham BM Phd (*Department of Health*)

In attendance

D. A. Pyke CBE MD FRCP (*Registrar*)

Linda Connah BA (*Deputy Secretary*)

Elaine M. Stephenson BA (*Working Party Secretary*)

Acknowledgements

The working party is grateful to the following for their advice:

Sir Richard Doll OBE DM FRCP FRCGP FRS (*Emeritus Professor of Medicine, University of Oxford*)

J. S. McCormick FRCP(I) FRCGP FFPHM (*Professor of Community Health, Trinity College, University of Dublin*)

Sir Philip Randle MD FRCP FRS (*Professor of Clinical Biochemistry, University of Oxford*)

A. J. Silman MD MRCP(UK) FFPHM (*Honorary Reader in Rheumatic Disease Epidemiology, University of Manchester*)

Figures and Tables taken from data supplied by the Office of Population Censuses and Surveys (OPCS), The Central Statistical Office and HMSO publications are reproduced by permission of the Controller of HMSO and are Crown copyright.

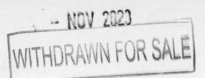
Preventive Medicine

*A report of a working party of the
Royal College of Physicians*

1991

ROYAL COLLEGE OF PHYSICIANS OF LONDON

The Royal College of Physicians
acknowledges the financial support
of this publication by
The Jerwood Foundation

Royal College of Physicians of London
11 St Andrew's Place, London NW1 4LE

Typeset by Oxprint Ltd, Aristotle Lane, Oxford OX2 6TR
Printed in Great Britain by Cathedral Press Ltd, Salisbury, Wilts

President's Statement

The prospects for action to prevent the development of many important diseases have much improved and have attracted increased and welcome attention in recent years. The current flood of information and opinion about preventive medicine has, however, made it difficult for non-specialists, both health professionals and laymen, to make reasoned judgements about this rapidly advancing field of medical knowledge.

In this Report the Royal College of Physicians gives an account of the current scope of preventive medicine. The Report especially aims to provide objective guidance about the factual content of often controversial topics, to assess the risks of different health problems for which preventive measures are proposed and the costs and benefits of preventive programmes. The Report also describes the practical steps which can be adopted by people generally and by health professionals to improve the prospects of good health in the community.

The Report is published at a particularly opportune time of intense discussion following publication of the Government's Green Paper 'The Health of the Nation'. We hope that the Report will help in facilitating informed discussion on many important issues which affect the health of us all.

MARGARET TURNER-WARWICK
President
Royal College of Physicians

November 1991

Format and scope of this report

After a preliminary chapter putting preventive medicine in the context of health care, each chapter of the report summarises current evidence about the major causes of disease, and discusses how it can be prevented. Emphasis is put on the contribution which doctors in clinical practice can make to prevention. Constraints on implementing preventive policies, which may be due to lack of knowledge, lack of organisation, lack of political will or lack of resources, are discussed.

Means of reducing the major life-style risks of smoking and alcohol are reviewed. The College has also produced detailed reports on these subjects: *Health or smoking* (1983) and *A great and growing evil: the medical consequences of alcohol abuse* (1987). In an Appendix, the economic consequences of limiting tobacco and alcohol consumption are also considered.

The role of diet to health is considered in a separate chapter as well as in the chapters on topics in which diet plays a part in prevention of disease.

The significant role of prevention in the reduction of some common diseases such as cancer, heart disease and stroke are discussed in some detail, as is the efficacy of screening.

Special attention is given to prevention of disease in children and in the elderly, and to prevention of infectious disease, accidents and occupational disease. The final chapter summarises the state of the art of preventive medicine based on current evidence of its effectiveness.

The references for each chapter are included in a reference section at the end of the book.

The report does not consider the prevention of mental illness or of addiction to drugs—other than alcohol and tobacco.

The increasing role of medical genetics in the prevention of inherited diseases is not specifically dealt with in this report, but was reviewed in an earlier College report *Prenatal diagnosis and genetic screening: community and service implications* (1989). The ethical issues raised in this area of medicine have also been addressed by the College.

HIV and other genito-urinary infections, although touched on in this report, are not dealt with extensively because of much recent coverage in the lay and technical literature and educational programmes already in existence.

Contents

1 Setting the scene

Historical perspective

The second half of the 19th century and first half of the 20th saw a dramatic fall in population mortality in the UK which was almost entirely attributable to the decline in deaths from infectious disease. During this period, various social and political changes led to better nutrition, better housing, better working conditions, better education and larger disposable income. Public health measures to improve the environment were introduced, most notably in the provision of a clean water supply and improved housing. Clinical interventions, such as immunisation and effective drug treatments for infection, came late in this period and so, in an historical perspective, their contribution to health has been relatively small. Hence, apart from doctors specialising in public health, the scope for preventive medicine in medical practice was small.

Present scope for preventive intervention

The main fatal conditions that afflict different age groups in the UK today are shown in Figs 1.1 and 1.2. As in times past, the distribution of disease reflects the hazards of the social and physical environment. Many hazards, such as availability of tobacco and alcohol, the increase in road traffic, social deprivation of inner city populations, unemployment and homelessness, whilst beyond the capacity of clinical medicine to alter, remain of prime concern to specialists in public health, and to the political voice of the medical profession as a whole. Superimposed upon these social and environmental factors, however, is the recognition that individuals can, by their own behaviour, reduce their risk of contracting disease, provided that they have the knowledge and incentive to do so. By increasing the understanding of the causes of many of the common serious diseases that now afflict developed societies, many possibilities are opened up for individuals to protect their own health.

There is now scope for preventive medicine to be fostered in the course of the clinical work of general practitioners and hospital doctors, as well as by those specialising in public health. Doctor–patient consultations provide opportunities for educating and advising patients about healthy life styles. Moreover, there is an increasing range of tests which can be used to screen for early detection of disease in order to avoid its

Fig. 1.1 *Deaths from all causes by age group, England and Wales, 1989. Source: OPCS.*

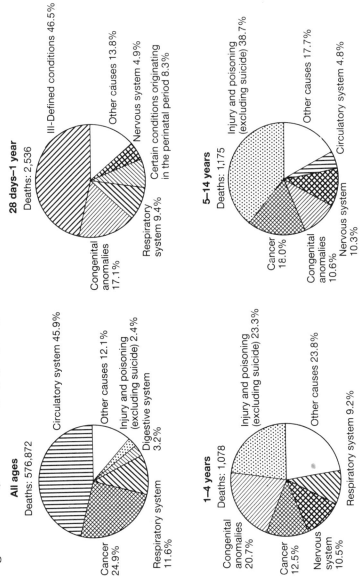

Fig. 1.1 *(continued)*

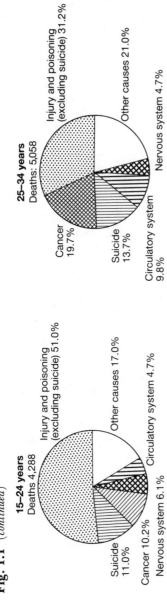

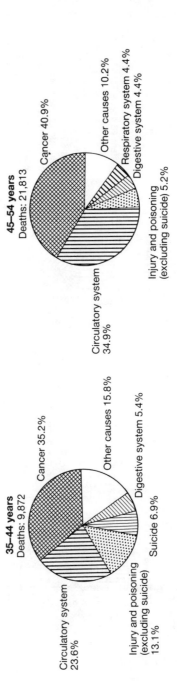

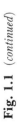
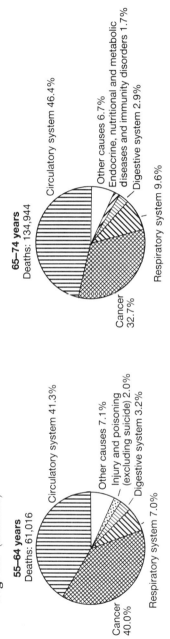
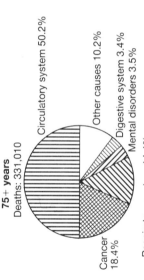

Fig. 1.1 (*continued*)

55–64 years
Deaths: 61,016

Circulatory system 41.3%

Other causes 7.1%

Injury and poisoning (excluding suicide) 2.0%

Digestive system 3.2%

Respiratory system 7.0%

Cancer 40.0%

65–74 years
Deaths: 134,944

Circulatory system 46.4%

Other causes 6.7%

Endocrine, nutritional and metabolic diseases and immunity disorders 1.7%

Digestive system 2.9%

Respiratory system 9.6%

Cancer 32.7%

75+ years
Deaths: 331,010

Circulatory system 50.2%

Other causes 10.2%

Digestive system 3.4%

Mental disorders 3.5%

Respiratory system 14.4%

Cancer 18.4%

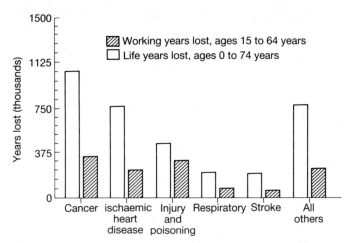

Fig. 1.2 *Life years and working years lost due to selected causes, England and Wales, 1987.* Source: *OPCS*.

full-blown consequences; and a greater range of vaccines and prophylactic drugs. Table 1.1 gives some examples of the wide range of activities that contribute to preventive medicine.

Definition of preventive medicine

The purpose of preventive medicine is

- to reduce the risk of a person contracting a disease, or
- by identifying an early manifestation of disease, to reduce the risk of subsequent disability or death.

The latter purpose merges into that of curative medicine where, for example, the management of a cigarette smoker who has had a myocardial infarct would include advice to stop smoking in order to lower the risk of a subsequent attack. Different levels of prevention are sometimes categorised as primary, secondary or tertiary:

- *primary prevention* aims at complete avoidance of the disease;
- *secondary prevention* aims at detecting and curing disease at a stage before it has caused any symptoms; and
- *tertiary prevention* aims at minimising the consequences for a patient who already has the disease.

In this report, 'preventive medicine' is taken to mean risk-reducing interventions targetted at 'well' individuals who are apparently free from the disease in question, ie primary and secondary prevention, although, particularly in the elderly, prevention of disability depends

Table 1.1   Examples of preventive activities

Type of prevention	Intervention	Responsibility for implementation
Statutory		
Reduction in cigarette smoking	Higher taxation	Government
Prevention of waterborne disease	Safe water supply	Water companies
Reduction of road traffic accidents	Breathalyser	Police
Reduction of childhood infections	Housing the homeless	Local authority
Prevention of foodborne disease	Inspection of food premises	Environmental health officers
Voluntary		
Reduction in cigarette smoking	Education in schools	Health promotion officers, school teachers
Reduction in coronary heart disease	Advice on reducing fat in diet	Doctors, health promotion officers, school teachers
Prevention of measles	Immunisation	Doctors
Reduction of invasive cervical cancer	Screening	Doctors

largely on recognition and treatment of symptoms which are already present (tertiary prevention). The report draws attention to those areas where political and legislative action may be needed in order to achieve control of a disease, but in the main it is focussed on describing the evidence on avoidable causes of disease, on the ways in which individuals can protect their own health, and on the ways in which clinical doctors can assist in this. In the recommendations, however, priority is given to legislative means of control in areas such as smoking, alcohol consumption and accidents where it is the view of the working party that this is the most powerful preventive strategy.

Evidence on the effectiveness of preventive medicine

On an international scale there are wide differences in various health indicators between countries of roughly similar development, and when examining time trends it can be seen that some countries have succeeded in reducing their rates of disease much more than others. Even within the UK there are wide variations in mortality and morbidity between different geographical regions and between different social classes.

These discrepancies lead to questions of why one country, region or class has better health than another, and what steps are needed to bring the worst up to the level of the best. For example, why has ischaemic heart disease mortality over the past 20 years declined by 50% in the US but only 25% in the UK? (see Chapter 5.) Part of the improvement may be due to better prevention and part to better treatment, but it is not always possible to identify the precise contribution made by each. Similar questions about why the UK has not done better are also applicable to diseases for which the aetiological agent has been clearly identified, such as lung cancer; or to diseases with long-established screening programmes of proven effectiveness such as cervical cancer; and until recently, to diseases for which immunisation of proven effectiveness is routinely available, such as measles.

To assess the effectiveness of a preventive strategy in reducing risk it is clearly necessary to define risk. We cannot predict with certainty whether an individual will or will not acquire a disease, but from the incidence rate in the population (the number of new cases of the disease per head of population in a defined time period) we can predict the probability of a person falling ill. For example, it is known that about two out of every 1000 60-year-old women will develop breast cancer each year; this means that the probability or risk for an individual woman is one in 500. Since risk can only be measured as probability, based on data from populations, so reduction in risk—or the effectiveness of prevention—can also only be quantified by population based studies. Prospective controlled trials of preventive activity are difficult and expensive, requiring large populations to be studied over lengthy time periods. It is therefore not surprising that there are still major gaps in our knowledge.

Epidemiological studies may have established risk factors for a specific disease, and by inference suggest that if the risk factor were eliminated the disease incidence would be reduced by a specified proportion; but demonstrating that reduction in practice is much more difficult and evidence is frequently lacking. Similarly, the prophylactic value of a drug in preventing deterioration or recurrence may have been established in patients who already have a disease, but its value as a preventive measure in those without manifest disease may be uncertain. Thus, three categories of *evidence of effectiveness* can be distinguished:

1. where experimental population-based trials have been carried out and have shown a specified level of risk reduction;

2. where there is strong evidence of benefit from non-experimental changes in population risk levels or from clinical treatment situations, but where population-based experimental trials have not been done; and

3. where risk factors are known but evidence on the effects of altering them is lacking.

In the past, some advances have been made by introducing measures without firm evidence of the size of benefit they would achieve or of their cost. Clinical preventive interventions such as immunisation or screening are amenable to formal experimental evaluation, but it is much harder to evaluate the effects of changes in life style.

Definition of risk

Perceptions of risk

There is often a wide gap between the perception of a particular health risk and the numerical risk as defined in terms of statistical probability. Common everyday personal health risks, such as crossing a road or smoking a cigarette, are greatly undervalued whereas rare environmental risks, particularly those not under the control of individuals such as non-occupational exposure to asbestos, are greatly overemphasised and often accompanied by political demands for preventive action. Similarly, although the statistical probability of a catastrophic event which kills or maims many people at once may be very low, such an event, particularly if it occurs close to home, provokes public fear and outrage out of all proportion to that expressed about common causes of disease or death. People also tend to underestimate the risks of activities they enjoy, such as smoking, drinking and dangerous sports. Doctors, being human, are not immune to distorted opinions of risk even in their own area of practice, and may tend to overemphasise the health risk or the health benefit of intervention without being able to put either in the context of total health risks. Where evidence is available, this report uses statistical estimates of risk reduction, although in many situations there is no direct evidence.

Measuring risk

The methods used to quantify risks in statistical terms are based on epidemiological information about the distribution of a disease in the population.

The risk of dying from any disease is readily available from routine mortality statistics compiled from death certificates. Each year the Office of Population Censuses and Surveys (OPCS) publishes tables which show how many people of a particular sex and age group die of a particular disease, and relates this to the number of people in that sex and age group in the population to give a mortality rate. For example, the annual mortality from accidents in young men aged 15–24 years is five per 10,000 indicating a risk of one in 2000 in each year for men in that age group. Over the 10-year period as a whole the *cumulative risk* is approximately 10 times greater, meaning that on his 15th birthday a youth has a one in 200 chance of dying from an accident before he is 25 years old.

For the purpose of evaluating primary prevention, it is preferable to know the incidence rate of new cases of the disease rather than the mortality rate, particularly for diseases which are not fatal but cause disability. But apart from cancers, congenital abnormalities and certain infectious diseases, there is no routine information system in the UK to record all new cases, and therefore incidence rates for many diseases can only be determined by special surveys. Often mortality data have to be used as a proxy for incidence data.

Risk factors

Comparisons of incidence and mortality rates in different time periods or different countries or population subgroups frequently generate hypotheses about specific aetiological agents or risk factors. Such hypotheses can then be further investigated to find out whether people who develop the disease have had more exposure to the risk factor than those who do not. Such investigations can either be done retrospectively by enquiring about past exposure in patients with the disease and in control subjects from the same background (case-control studies); or prospectively by measuring the prevalence of exposure to the risk factor in a population and keeping track of them all to find out which individuals subsequently develop disease (cohort studies). Both methods enable estimation of the *relative risk*, ie the risk of an exposed person relative to that of an unexposed person.

A relative risk of two means that a person exposed to the risk factor is twice as likely to get the disease as a person who has not been exposed. But an increased relative risk on its own does not indicate what the actual level of risk is for such a person; the latter depends also on the underlying risk in the non-exposed. For example, it now seems clear that use of oral contraceptives (OC) at young ages and before first pregnancy leads to an increased risk of developing breast cancer before the age of 45, relative to OC non-users, of about 50% (relative

risk 1.5). But because the incidence of breast cancer below age 45 is in
any case low, this only translates to a change from one in 500 risk of
developing breast cancer before age 45 in non-users to a one in 300 risk
for OC users. (Risk is related also to duration of use of OCs—see
Chapter 6.)

The prospective method of measuring risk also measures the rate of
the disease in exposed people and in unexposed. The difference between
these two rates is the *attributable risk* which is a measure of the rate of
disease associated with the risk factor, and thus indicates how much
disease could be prevented by eliminating exposure. The size of the
attributable risk depends both on the prevalence of exposure to the risk
factor and the size of the relative risk. If either, or both, of these are
low the attributable risk will be small. If both are large, as in the
example of smoking and lung cancer (see Chapter 2) the attributable
risk, and hence the potential for health gain from prevention, will be
large.

Drawbacks of preventive medicine

A particular ethical responsibility rests on doctors who offer preventive
interventions to be certain that the benefits of what they are offering
outweigh its disadvantages. This is because they are advising an
outwardly healthy person rather than a patient with declared disease,
and they must therefore have evidence that the probability of a health
gain far exceeds the probability of physical, psychological or social
disadvantage. One of the dangers of preventive medicine is that it may
needlessly turn some well people into people who feel ill, the 'worried
well', or may actually cause iatrogenic disease. For example, there may
be unwanted side effects of a vaccine; a screening programme may give
false positive results; or treatment of a symptomless condition may
have side effects which themselves cause unpleasant symptoms. It is
often exceedingly difficult to balance the net health effect of a large
number of people who are caused minor morbidity against a small
number of people in whom major morbidity is avoided. The doctor
must not only be certain in his own mind that the balance is in favour
of the preventive intervention, but should also do all he can to ensure
that the people he is advising themselves understand the risks and the
benefits.

Cost-effectiveness of preventive activity

Resources for health creation (by prevention or treatment) are finite
and cannot be sufficient to meet all the demands made on them.

Acknowledging scarcity means accepting that a recommendation to direct resources to any preventive measure involves forgoing benefits which could have been gained elsewhere. 'Cost' is thus perceived in terms of the sacrifices involved in pursuing the prevention programme rather than solely in terms of the money spent on the programme itself.

An efficient programme is one which maximises reductions in morbidity and mortality within available resources, although considerations other than efficiency, such as equity and consumer preference, also need to be taken into account in formulating policy. On the basis of the efficiency criterion, however, the generally accepted rule that no programme should be recommended if it does more harm than good, is enlarged to include rejection when small potential benefits can be realised only at very high cost, ie larger health gains can be achieved by using these resources in other programmes.

Moreover, costs and benefits can vary markedly as programmes are expanded or contracted. Thus a small scale programme targetted only at high risk groups may be recommended, while a larger programme to include lower risk groups may not be justified by the high cost of achieving these marginal benefits. This principle applies to frequency of intervention as well as size of target populations, for example annual versus five-yearly screening. Implicit in such policy decisions is the fact that they are based on current practice. Any improvement in the efficiency of a programme, say by technological innovation or the discovery of more cost-effective ways of providing the service, will require a re-assessment of the marginal costs and benefits of the policy.

There is a widespread belief that, because it reduces the need for high cost treatment, prevention is cheaper than cure but this is not necessarily true. In the case of primary prevention, the cost of reducing the risk of the entire population can be higher than the cost of treating the cases which arise in the absence of prevention. With secondary prevention, the cost of screening the entire at-risk population plus the cost of presymptomatic treatment of those detected, can be much higher than the resource cost of treating cases as they become symptomatic. Added to this, of course, those who do not succumb to the condition may later make additional demands on health care resources. This long-term consequence of effective intervention applies equally to treatment as well as prevention, and cannot be used as a valid argument against the intervention. The spurious argument that early death is beneficial to the economy is discussed in the Appendix.

The fact that a prevention programme does not save resources in no way implies that prevention should not be actively pursued. There are many situations in treatment as well as prevention, in which it would be cheaper to let people die rather than prolong their lives. As with any health care programme, the objective of prevention is to achieve health gains by a reduction in morbidity and mortality and these are achieved at a cost. The benefits of such reductions come in many forms including less pain and suffering, more mobility, and longer life, in addition to any benefits in the form of resource savings. Given the scarcity of resources and the perception of cost as sacrifice, a preventive measure is justified if the value of all these benefits is greater than the costs of achieving them. **Thus, an efficient programme is not one which saves money but one in which the sum of all benefits exceeds the sum of all costs**.

The decision as to whether benefits, in terms of years of life gained or improved quality of life, are 'worth' the cost of achieving them is, of course, a value judgement but the need to make such value judgements is inescapable. Health benefits cannot be 'above considerations of cost' or 'of infinite value'; it should always be remembered that they can only be achieved at the sacrifice of benefits elsewhere. Only in a world of infinite resources would the above two quotations be true. This is not to say, of course, that there is no scope for debate on how much of the national resources are devoted to health in relation to other demands. It is also important to remember that many other aspects of the economy, such as education, employment, housing, transport and agricultural policy, have important influences on the health of a population. While doctors and economists can provide expert views on the consequences of different preventive policies, the size of the health budget is the responsibility of government, and the allocation of priorities within the Health Service is the responsibility of the health authorities. The value judgement of a health authority on the preventive policy which will maximise health gain for its entire population may well differ from that of a clinical doctor whose responsibility is to maximise health gain for the individual patient consulting him. For example, the health authority may wish to use any available resource for improving uptake of screening by previously unscreened people, rather than increasing the frequency of screening. Whereas the clinical doctor may see maximum health gain for his patient by screening more frequently. Conflicts therefore arise when clinical doctors wish to apply a preventive action for their individual patients' benefit but government and health authority policy has not made money available for this purpose.

2 Smoking

History of smoking

The habit of smoking dried leaves of tobacco (*Nicotiana tabacum*) was known to the North American Indians for centuries before Christopher Columbus landed in America but he was blamed for having introduced the habit to Spain in the 16th century. From Spain, smoking quickly spread to other European countries.[1] Sir Walter Raleigh is said to have introduced it to Britain where Queen Elizabeth I was quick to realise its revenue potential by imposing the first tobacco tax of two-pence in the pound. In 1604, her successor, James I, wrote a violent diatribe against smoking entitled *A Counterblaste to Tobacco* in which he described tobacco as: 'hateful to the nose, harmful to the brain and dangerous to the lungs'; but even he recognised the seductive nature of the habit and the extraordinary paradoxical psychological effects of nicotine: 'being taken when they go to bed, it makes one sleepe soundly, and yet being taken when a man is sleepie and drowsie, it will, as they say, awake his braine and quicken his understanding.' During the 17th century tobacco consumption increased in Britain, when it was smoked mostly in pipes but also chewed and, in fashionable circles, used as snuff.

The first cigarettes were made in the mid-18th century in Brazil and afterwards found their way to mainland Europe from where they were introduced to Britain by soldiers returning from the Crimean War. However, it was the production of milder Virginia tobaccos and the development of the briar pipe which further boosted tobacco smoking in the 19th century. The development of improved flue-curing of tobacco and the mechanisation of cigarette manufacture (replacing hand-rolled cigarettes) at the end of the 19th century, finally set the scene for the huge increase in tobacco smoking in developed countries in the last 50 years or so, and the current escalation in the Third World. The consequent epidemic of smoking-related disease and premature death has now become a worldwide phenomenon.

Smoking prevalence

The proportion of men in the population in Britain who smoke reached a peak at the end of the Second World War when almost two-thirds of men were smoking; in women this peak occurred about a quarter of a

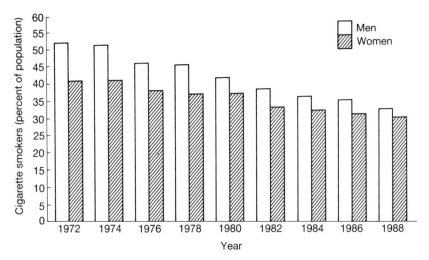

Fig. 2.1 *Percentage of population who smoked cigarettes, by sex, England and Wales 1972 to 1988.* Source: *OPCS*[2].

century later, in the 1970s, when over 40% of all women smoked cigarettes. Since then, cigarette smoking has been declining in both sexes and all age groups, but the decline has been less steep in women than in men (Fig. 2.1). In young women there seems to have been little or no decline in recent years. In 1988, 33% of men and 30% of women were cigarette smokers.[2]

Social class

Until about 1960, smoking was more or less equally common in all social classes. Since then a steep socio-economic gradient in smoking prevalence has developed so that by 1988 only about one in six of professional men and women were smoking compared with about two in five men and women in the lowest socio-economic group (Fig. 2.2).

Children

Tobacco smoking by children continues to cause serious concern. Many children experiment with smoking at an early age and boys tend to do so earlier than girls; in 1988, 17% of boys compared with 12% of girls had tried smoking by the time they were 11 years old. However, girls catch up later on, and overtake boys so that by the time they are 14 years, boys and girls are equally likely to have tried smoking. Older girls are more likely to have done so than boys. Encouragingly,

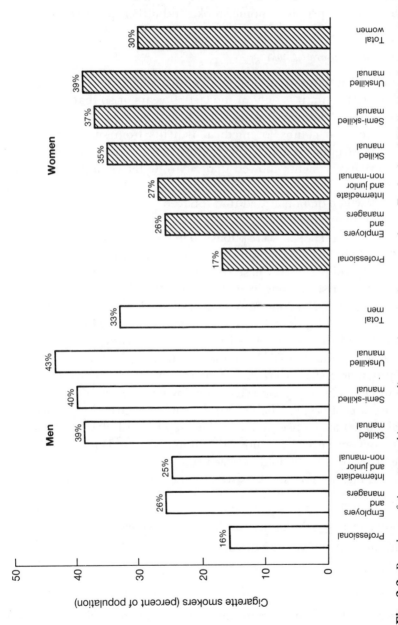

Fig. 2.2 *Prevalence of cigarette smoking according to socio-economic group and sex, England and Wales 1988. Source: OPCS[2]*

however, the proportion of regular smokers (at least one cigarette a week) in the 11–15 year age group has declined in recent years and in 1988 was 7% in boys and 9% in girls, with about a fifth of these smoking ten cigarettes a day. Children are much more likely to be smokers if other people at home smoke and if their peers smoke.

Health consequences of smoking

Although King James I, almost four centuries ago, viewed smoking as injurious to health, it is only in the last 30 years or so that irrefutable evidence of the damage it causes has been obtained. In the interim, there were even claims for medical benefits from smoking—in the treatment of gout, stomach ulcers and even cancer! In the 1930s, laboratory experiments showed that cigarette tar could produce skin cancer in animals, but it was the epidemiological studies initiated in the 1940s which demonstrated that tobacco smoking greatly increases the risk of lung cancer.

In 1950, several papers were published in the UK and USA comparing the smoking habits of large numbers of patients with lung cancer with those of control patients. These studies suggested that heavy smoking increased the risk of lung cancer up to 30-fold[3,4] and the findings provoked further research on the effect of smoking on mortality. The smoking habits of large cohorts of men and women were elicited and recorded, and the causes of death of those subsequently dying were ascertained. Numerous large studies of this type all showed higher mortality amongst smokers than non-smokers; this was especially true of cigarette smoking; pipe and cigar smoking were only weakly associated with increased mortality. This research included such classical epidemiological studies as the twenty-year follow-up of British doctors[5,6] and the American Cancer Society study of 1 million people.[7] Differences in risk of the order of 10 to 20 fold between smokers of 20 or more cigarettes daily and lifelong non-smokers were found for:

- lung cancer
- some cancers of the upper respiratory and digestive tracts
- chronic obstructive lung disease
- right heart failure
- aortic aneurysm.

Smaller, but highly significant, differences were found for death from some other cancers, ischaemic heart disease, and peptic ulcer.[8,5] These studies also showed that stopping smoking was associated with a decline in mortality.

Additional hazards for women

For women, smoking poses additional hazards. These include:

- increased risk of vascular disease associated with oral contraceptive use
- increased risk of carcinoma of cervix
- in pregnancy, increased risk of miscarriage, premature fetal death and retarded physical and mental development of the baby
- an earlier menopause, and an increased risk of osteoporosis and bone fractures.

Size of the problem

In 1962, the Royal College of Physicians published the first of its four Reports on smoking and health.[9] This report concluded that cigarette smoking now presented the most challenging opportunity for preventive medicine, and was as important a cause of death in modern times as were the great epidemic diseases of the past such as typhoid, cholera and tuberculosis.

In the most recent of its four reports on smoking,[10] the Royal College of Physicians estimated that tobacco smoking accounted for 15–20% of all deaths in Britain, a total of at least 100,000 deaths a year. In today's terms, for the UK this includes:

- at least 90% of the approximately 40,000 lung cancer deaths
- three-quarters of the approximately 20,000 deaths from chronic obstructive lung disease
- a quarter of the approximately 180,000 coronary heart disease deaths.

The following statements[11] graphically illustrate the mortality attributable to smoking:

- About a quarter of all regular smokers of 20 or more cigarettes will be killed early by their smoking.
- Some of these would have lived ten, twenty or even thirty years more.
- On average those killed by smoking will lose ten to fifteen years of life.

Taking an average 1,000 young men in Britain, who regularly smoke 20 or more cigarettes daily, about:

- One will be murdered
- Six will be killed on the roads
- 250 will be killed by tobacco.

Peto further estimated that of all deaths in middle-age, about one-third are tobacco-related. The death toll from smoking in the UK provides the familiar analogy of a jumbo jet crashing each day with the loss of life of all on board.

Passive (involuntary) smoking

In recent years, there has been increasing concern about 'passive smoking' and it now seems clear that the harmful effects of smoking are not confined to the smoker.[12] This issue has become more prominent as the size of the non-smoking majority in the population has increased, and as other sources of environmental pollution have diminished.

Early epidemiological studies showed that children in households where parents smoke had more respiratory tract infections than those in non-smoking households.[13] Others had shown impairment of respiratory function in adults working in smoky environments.[14] However, the main concern has been about the possible carcinogenic effects of passive smoking. Over 20 epidemiological studies have now investigated this by observing lung cancer rates in the non-smoking spouses of people who do, or do not, smoke.[15] Most of them have demonstrated that non-smokers who have been exposed to passive smoking have an increased risk of lung cancer relative to other non-smokers in the range 10–50% (relative risk 1.1 to 1.5). This means that people who haver never smoked but who have been regularly exposed to environmental tobacco smoke through most of their lives have about a 30% higher risk of lung cancer than non-smokers not so exposed. It suggests that several hundred lung cancer deaths in the UK each year in non-smokers are due to this cause.[12]

The smoking habit

Initiation into smoking almost invariably starts in childhood, and puberty seems to be a critical point for acquiring the habit. Parents, siblings and the peer group all play an important role. Having a parent who smokes increases the youngster's likelihood of smoking; both parents being smokers increases this further, as does having an elder brother or sister who smokes. But the greatest influence comes from friends of a similar age. In one study, over half the adolescents who smoked had friends who also smoked compared with only one in seven of non-smokers.

Initially, smoking is adopted in spite of, rather than because of, the effect of nicotine and the first experience of smoking is usually unpleasant, often causing feelings of dizziness, nausea and vomiting. But because of the social influences causing its initiation, the habit is persisted with and tolerance to nicotine develops. The unpleasant pharmacological effects then disappear, being replaced in many smokers by nicotine dependence.[16]

Inhalation of tobacco smoke results in remarkably efficient delivery of nicotine to the brain, the interval between inhalation and the onset of nicotine's action on the brain being less than 10 seconds. Repetition of the process many times with each cigarette (and several hundred times a day for the average smoker) ensures regularly repeated 'shots' of the drug. Dependence is thus reinforced with a frequency very much greater than that associated with injectable drugs of addiction such as heroin.

But pharmacological addiction to nicotine is not the only or complete explanation for persistence of smoking. The apparatus and activities associated with smoking may be helpful in stressful situations and, although the social acceptability of smoking is now declining, the offering and acceptance of cigarettes has long been an acknowledged way of mediating and facilitating social interaction. Stopping smoking involves coping with the difficulty of changing deeply ingrained habits as well as with withdrawal from drug dependency.

Helping people to stop smoking (See also Appendix to this Chapter)

The relationship between smoking and disease is now universally accepted, but many smokers think the risk is confined to 'heavy smokers' and especially underestimate the risk of heart disease. They also doubt the benefits of stopping, feeling that the damage has already been done, and being generally fatalistic. Even so, most adults who smoke say they want to stop smoking and have made attempts to do so. Amongst ex-smokers, most have achieved this status without any special help and the majority also seem to find it easier than they expected, though a substantial minority, especially heavy smokers, do seem to find it very difficult.

Only about one-third of smokers acknowledge having been advised by doctors to stop smoking, but most claim they would make a serious attempt to stop if advised to do so by their doctors.[17]

Role of health professionals

Health professionals have an important exemplar role and this is especially true of doctors, the great majority of whom are now non-smokers. Only about 12% of general practitioners still smoke, and fewer than half of them smoke cigarettes.[18]

The potential for doctors, especially in primary care, to advise about smoking is considerable. Patients expect their doctors to ask and advise about their lifestyle, including smoking habits,[19] and this activity is now part of the 'Terms of Service' of general practitioners under their 1990 NHS Contract. There is also evidence that patients attach particular significance to the advice of a personal doctor.[20]

There is good evidence that the advice of general practitioners helps patients to stop smoking. Randomised trials have shown that minimal intervention—simple advice supplemented with a leaflet—as an incidental part of a normal general practice consultation, can achieve a one-year sustained cessation rate of about 5%.[21,22] Higher success rates have been achieved with more intensive interventions, including the use of nicotine chewing gum, and in clinics where support and follow-up is maintained.[23] Furthermore, general practitioner advice to stop smoking is very cost effective, more so than other measures of coronary heart disease prevention such as controlling hypertension, lowering plasma cholesterol, or carrying out coronary artery bypass surgery.[24,25]

Because simple advice achieves a small but significant level of sustained smoking cessation, such advice should be routinely included in all general practice consultations with smokers. Likewise, hospital doctors should use every opportunity, in both outpatient and inpatient settings, to advise those patients who smoke to stop.

Just asking patients about smoking indicates the health significance of the habit, and smoking enquiry and advice must be part of any consultation concerned with:

    Respiratory complaints
    Smoking-related diseases
    Diabetes
    Hypertension
    Oral contraception
    Pregnancy
    Forthcoming operations

Parents consulting with young children who have respiratory infections should be asked about their own smoking habits and the opportunity used to point out the harmful effect of parental smoking on the health of children.

The general practice potential for reducing smoking prevalence

General practice is uniquely placed for giving advice on lifestyle. The average general practitioner has a list of about 2,000 patients. Of the 1,500 or so who are over the age of 16 years, about one-third, ie 500, will be smokers, and at least two-thirds will consult at least once a year (smokers do so more often than others). If 5% of smokers stop permanently after receiving simple advice, giving this on one occasion only to all smokers who consult a GP during the course of a year could achieve 15–20 ex-smokers a year. **Collectively, general practitioners could help about half a million patients a year to stop smoking.**[21] If this seems an extravagant claim, it should be remembered that about a quarter of a million patients who smoke cross the thresholds of general practice surgeries each day and many patients expect lifestyle inquiry and advice when they do so.

Smoking and the workplace

Recognition of the harmful effects of involuntary smoking[11] has stimulated anti-smoking activities in the working environment. This has included the introduction of policies restricting smoking in places of work (an employer is obliged to provide a healthy and safe working environment), and provision of help for smokers wanting to stop. Occupational health services therefore now have increasing opportunities to involve themselves in offering advice on stopping smoking, as well as the identification and management of other risk factors (see also Appendix B to this chapter).

Educating school-children about smoking

In recent years there has been a major expansion of health education in the school curriculum and this has included information and advice about smoking. A survey of 11–15 year olds in 1988 showed that about half remembered having at least one lesson about smoking; the proportion ranged from about one-quarter of first year secondary school pupils to about two-thirds of those in the final year.[29] In 1989 the Health Education Authority, with government support, launched a major five-year programme aimed at persuading teenagers not to smoke. This campaign includes not only national advertising but also support for educational programmes run by local education authorities and health authorities.

Recommended political actions to control smoking

The Royal College of Physicians, together with many other organisations such as the World Health Organisation and International Union Against Cancer, have made recommendations about the control of tobacco to reduce the disease, disability and premature death which it causes. Measures which have been consistently recommended include:

- Stopping all forms of promotion of tobacco products
- Raising price through taxation
- Public information and education programmes
- Strong, prominent health warnings on packs
- Controlling smoking in public places
- Banning sales to children
- Reducing tar content of cigarettes.

Voluntary agreements

'Voluntary agreements' between government and the tobacco industry have a limited usefulness. Legislation is required to implement most of these measures effectively. The economic consequences of curtailing cigarette smoking are fully discussed in the Appendix to this report (p 200) which concludes that, provided smoking prevalence falls in a gradual fashion, the national economy need not suffer and the health of the country would be vastly improved.

RECOMMENDATIONS

1   All forms of promotion of tobacco products should be prohibited.

2   Price rises of tobacco products should exceed the rate of inflation to discourage increasing sales.

3   Legislation prohibiting tobacco sales to children should be enforced.

4   Restrictions on smoking in public places and workplaces should be extended.

5   Public education, including that in the school curriculum, about the importance of tobacco as a major risk to health should be maintained and enhanced.

6   All health professionals should offer smoking cessation advice in any consultation with smokers.

7 Health professionals should emphasise avoidance of smoking as a priority issue.

8 Medical education should ensure doctors are well-equipped to inform and advise patients about tobacco smoking.

9 More support services should be available to help those involved in smoking cessation work.

10 Research on more effective ways to stop smoking should be conducted.

11 On all health-care premises, non-smoking should be the norm and tobacco sales should be prohibited.

12 A tobacco levy could provide resources for public education about tobacco.

Appendix

A. STOPPING SMOKING

Suggestions for what and how to advise

The Stages

There is no simple 'prescription' for stopping smoking and success is associated with a variety of approaches; the most effective help is likely to be personalised to the needs of the individual concerned. In giving advice it is important to acknowledge that stopping smoking is a process, not a single event, and it may be helpful to identify *four basic stages* in this:

1. Thinking about stopping
2. Deciding and preparing to stop
3. Actually stopping
4. Permanently abstaining.

1. Thinking about stopping

Intention to give up and confidence in the likelihood of doing so are good predictors of success.[17] Motivation to stop may be enhanced by information from mass media, public campaigns, tobacco tax increases, restriction on smoking in public places, social pressures, and so on. But advice and support from health professionals is a key element because of its personal nature.

Recording in medical records whether or not a patient smokes is an essential ingredient of medical care and can be facilitated by the use of special stickers, risk factor record cards, or a rubber stamp. Inquiry about interest in stopping and about the smoker's own reasons for wishing to do so should then follow. Positive reasons which emphasise the benefits of stopping, such as improvements in breathing, reduced susceptibility to illness, and social and financial gains, are likely to enhance motivation.

2. Deciding and preparing to stop

For some, stopping smoking may be suddenly provoked by personal illness or smoking-related illness or death of a close relative or friend. But for others, a strategy and plan may be devised which could include:

- Choosing a 'stopping day'. This may need to be some way ahead, or associated with an event such as New Year's Day or National No Smoking Day.
- Involving a spouse or close friend to increase commitment.
- Planning how to cope with smoking situations and danger times such as tea breaks, after meals, having a drink etc.
- Use of self-help literature providing guidelines.

3. Actually stopping

Stopping completely rather than attempting to do so gradually is generally best. But cutting out 'less essential' cigarettes, preparatory to actually stopping, may sometimes be helpful. A 'day at a time' approach should be adopted. Having something to nibble, suck or chew may be helpful and the support of friends and colleagues is vital.

4. Permanently abstaining

'Staying stopped' is the ultimate aim. The difficult stage is the early days and weeks, and, although some do find this period very difficult, others may find it relatively easy. The support and encouragement of a health professional, especially a general practitioner or practice nurse, may be particularly valuable at this stage in helping to prevent relapse. Even if stopping was easy, relapse may occur. As Mark Twain claimed 'Quitting smoking is easy; I've done it hundreds of times!'

Summary of advice

- Raising the issue
- Recording smoking habits in medical records
- Inquiring about interest in giving up
- Giving information and advice about stopping
- Helping to plan a strategy for stopping
- Offering a leaflet, follow-up and support
- Helping non-smokers not to start and ex-smokers not to relapse

B. ADDITIONAL AIDS TO STOPPING SMOKING
The relative merits of other aids to stopping smoking are set out below

1. Leaflets

The most useful adjunct to advice is a simple leaflet on how to stop smoking. Such leaflets are available from the Health Education Authority (Hamilton House, Mabledon Place, London WC1) and several other organisations.

2. Nicotine chewing gum

Although acquisition of the smoking habit is largely determined by social and psychological factors, dependence on the pharmacological effects of nicotine becomes a dominant influence for many smokers, and for this reason there is interest in alternative sources of nicotine as an aid to stopping smoking. Nicotine chewing gum was introduced to Britain for this purpose in 1980; it is not available on the NHS.

Several trials have demonstrated the efficacy of nicotine chewing gum in giving up smoking but the evidence has largely come from special smoking cessation clinics which recruit smokers who are highly motivated to stop and provide intensive and sustained interventions which may not be practicable in everyday medical settings. The evidence of efficacy of nicotine chewing gum in general practice is not very convincing, probably because of the relatively casual way in which it is prescribed and supervised.[26]

Its effectiveness depends on proper use, and careful instruction is therefore important. Chewing the gum releases nicotine which is absorbed through the lining of the mouth. A piece of gum should be used whenever the urge to smoke is strong and it should be chewed slowly and intermittently. Incorrect chewing technique may result in soreness of the mouth or throat, hiccups, or indigestion. If found helpful, use of the gum should be continued for three or four months, after which time most people are able to wean themselves off it (but a few are unable to do so). Two strengths are available: 2 mg and 4 mg. Individuals vary in the number of pieces they need but the average is usually about ten daily. It should not be used in pregnancy, by nursing mothers, or by those with peptic ulcers. Nicotine nasal spray and skin patches are currently being tested and are likely to become available in due course.

3. Carbon monoxide (CO) meter

The development of small, portable, reasonably cheap carbon monoxide meters has provided an instrument ('Smokerlyser') which may be helpful as an anti-smoking aid. Demonstrating the carbon monoxide concentration in expired breath may be a way of increasing motivation and helping patients to stop and there is some evidence that this works.[22]

4. Other methods

Provided it is not harmful, any other method a smoker wishes to try in an effort to stop smoking should not be discouraged. A desire to stop, confidence in the ability to do so, and belief in a method are crucial factors in success. Endorsement of this belief may therefore be valuable.

Such other methods include hypnosis and acupuncture which some smokers undoubtedly find helpful in enabling them to stop but which have not so far been shown by a scientific evaluation to have a specific effect. Promotion of methods should, however, be limited to those of proven effectiveness; exaggerated claims for methods of unproven effectiveness may reduce credibility and be counter-productive.

5. Smokers' clinics

So-called 'smokers clinics' are for smokers who have decided they want to stop smoking, need help in doing so and feel that the group setting of a smokers clinic may help them. Disappointingly, few such clinics have evaluated the outcome of their activities and they have been criticised[27] because of their very limited role in helping smokers to stop. To match the potential of UK general practice in this role about 10,000 smokers clinics would need to be available! But this criticism underestimates the potential role of such clinics as an identifiable base which could provide support at a local level for all activities concerned with stopping smoking; they are an important research base and could provide training, advice and support for health professionals as well as resources such as patient literature.[28]

6. Advice on stopping smoking in the workplace

ASH: Action on Smoking and Health (109 Gloucester Place, London W1H 3PH) operates a consultancy service which advises employers on implementing policies on smoking in the workplace.
QUIT (102 Gloucester Place, London W1H 3DA) also provides smoking cessation courses in the workplace.

3 Alcohol

Many people enjoy the taste of alcoholic drinks and the agreeable change of mood that comes with drinking in moderation. But alcohol is a potentially dangerous and addictive drug, and many people who have been damaged by its misuse were unaware of its dangers. Misuse of alcohol causes enormous fiscal damage to the nation and to individuals and also causes much social disruption, morbidity and mortality.* The Office of Health Economics estimated a loss of 8–15 million days a year in Great Britain because of alcohol misuse,[1] whilst an estimate of the minimum financial cost to England and Wales in 1983 was £1,614.5 million,[2] but it might be several times higher. The estimate was the sum of factors that included lost productivity, increased consumption of medical and social support, and legal expenses. Against this must be set a revenue of £6,000 million from duty, exports, and employment of 250,000 people (see Appendix).

Social damage

Family

Social damage caused by alcohol misuse pervades the family[8] and society at large. Although family problems are often multifactorial, a survey of divorces suggested that, in 30%, alcohol was an important contributory factor. In a survey of 100 battered women, 52 said that alcohol had played a significant role and in a recent survey of women admitted to hospital after an overdose of drugs, a third complained that their husbands were heavy drinkers. Constant arguments, violence, and emotional and physical deprivation readily affect the children of such families whose problems may present initially as a poor school work record or a change in behaviour. The more general social effects

---

*This report contains a relatively brief account of alcohol, not because it is unimportant— it is profoundly important—but because in 1987 The Royal College of Physicians produced a full report on alcohol abuse entitled *A Great and Growing Evil*.[3] Moreover four other reports have recently been published from professional medical bodies in the UK, namely *Alcohol, our favourite drug* (Royal College of Psychiatrists, 1986),[4] *Alcohol, a balanced view* (Royal College of General Practitioners, 1986),[5] *ABC of Alcohol* (British Medical Association, 1988),[6] and *Alcohol and the Public Health* (Faculty of Public Health Medicine, 1991).[7] These documents each give a thorough review of the subject and contain a comprehensive bibliography.

of alcohol misuse include occupational incompetence,[9] drunken driving,[10] criminal activity[11] and finally descent to skid row and homelessness.

Occupation

Certain occupations, such as those in the drink industry, catering, deep sea fishing and journalism, have a high incidence of alcohol misuse; the reasons are not completely clear but availability of cheap alcohol, isolated living conditions and group culture all play a part. Until recently, the medical profession was in this group; in 1970 the standardised mortality ratio (SMR) for cirrhosis of the liver among medical practitioners was 311. More recent figures[12] show a downward trend with an SMR of 115, ie a 15% excess mortality compared to the general population.

Excessive drinking can lead to:

- time off work
- incompetence in the form of poor decision making or personal relationships
- accidents.

Accidents may be due to the effects of high blood alcohol—either from drinking at work or the night before, or the effects of a hangover. By arranging for an employee to have a less onerous job or to take early retirement, the extent of alcohol misuse may be disguised in the work place. Few studies have been undertaken on the role of alcohol and accidents at work, but a survey in France[13] showed that alcohol was present in the blood in 35% of workers who had experienced accidents and 30% were chronic drinkers. Alcohol misuse may also lead to repeated dismissals, a gradual sliding down the skills ladder and finally to permanent unemployment.

Crime

Crime, including serious crime, is related to alcohol misuse.[11] In a review of 18 studies on homicide, more than half the offenders had been drinking at the time the offence was committed. An American study of 77 convicted rapists showed that half of them had been drinking before the offence was committed,[14] while a significant correlation was found when trends in violent deaths in Norway were plotted, including accidents, against changing consumption of alcohol. Other studies have shown alcohol consumption to be associated with burglary and violent behaviour, including that of patients in hospital casualty departments. It is probable that alcohol gives the criminal Dutch courage before a premeditated act, while impaired judgement after alcohol makes criminal activities more likely.

Accidents

It has been estimated that alcohol was an important factor in a third of all home accidents and in 26% of fatal accidents in the home; it was also associated with 26% of deaths from drowning.

Society is now well aware of the relationship between drinking and driving accidents[10] because of advertising campaigns and legislation — and often because of the death of a friend or relative. The Road Traffic Act of 1967 made it illegal to drive in Great Britain with a blood alcohol level greater than 80 mg%. The level was based on evidence such as that given in the Grand Rapids Survey in the USA which found that drivers with blood alcohol levels greater than 80 mg/100 ml had an increased risk of accidents which rose steeply when levels of 100 mg/100 ml were exceeded. In 1981, there were 63,832 convictions for drinking and driving in England and Wales. When this is set against a survey estimating that only one in 250 suspected offenders was convicted, the problem is seen to be enormous.[15]

Conversely, a high proportion of those injured in road accidents had been drinking. In a study of fatal motor accidents, 31% of the drivers had been drinking as had 29% of the passengers, and 21% of pedestrians killed in such accidents.

The increased risk of accidents is greater in young drivers and in frequent drinkers. This is of especial importance for it appears that drinking among young people has increased.[16]

Psychiatric factors

Psychiatric disorders may be the cause of, or the result of, alcohol misuse.[3,4] At first, alcohol lightens the mood and releases anxiety and so may give false confidence to cope with stresses at home or work, or to undertake unlawful and criminal acts. Gradually, the personality may change to become boastful, dogmatic and rather silly, and eventually it may deteriorate permanently. Frequent heavy drinking may be followed by amnesia for the event next day. Persistent drinkers often need a drink the following morning to steady their nerves and tremor and eventually delirium tremens may ensue. Other psychiatric disorders are hallucinosis, morbid jealousy and dementia. Misuse of alcohol is associated with abuse of other drugs, including tobacco.

Physical effects

The popular conception of liver disease as the main physical disability caused by alcohol abuse is false. No system of the body is immune and the vulnerable system(s) which will bear the brunt of the toxicity cannot be predicted for any individual. Thus, any of the conditions listed in Table 3.1 may occur in isolation or in unpredictable combination. The commonest presenting abnormalities are abnormal blood tests found on routine testing, such as raised mean red blood cell volume (MCV) and abnormal liver function tests, while the commonest disorders are intoxication, blackouts with resultant injuries, tremors and fits, liver disease, morning nausea, diarrhoea, infertility, raised blood pressure and pancreatitis. The metabolic basis for the varied susceptibility of different organs and systems between individuals is not yet understood. Alcohol intake during pregnancy can lead to babies with low birth weight, mental retardation and under-development of the mid-face (the fetal alcohol syndrome). Modest alcohol consumption seems to protect against coronary artery disease. In several studies people with a low alcohol consumption have been found to have a lower risk of coronary heart disease than complete abstainers[17] (see also Chapter 5). High levels of consumption increase the risk of coronary heart disease possibly by inducing hypertension.

PREVENTION

The litany of fiscal burdens, social ills and medical disabilities induced or aggravated by alcohol misuse leaves little doubt that great efforts must be made to reduce the damage. How can this be achieved? The aim of any prevention policy in a Western culture is reduction of intake and not prohibition, which is unacceptable to society. The aim is to cut down the overall intake of alcohol by the nation, with specific emphasis on vulnerable groups and risky situations. The rationale for aiming to cut down overall national consumption is based on the work of Ledermann.[18] Using deaths from cirrhosis as the most accessible marker of alcoholic damage, he showed a strong correlation between deaths from cirrhosis and alcohol consumption per head when various countries were compared. Repeated comparison under different circumstances (Fig. 3.1) has confirmed his findings.[19] This type of relationship also holds when alcohol consumption varies within a country; for example, in Britain alcohol consumption doubled between 1950 and 1980 and so did cirrhosis deaths, and as consumption rose between 1970 and 1984 so did the various social and medical consequences[4] (Table 3.2).

Table 3.1 Summary of medical health hazards associated with alcohol abuse *Source*: Ref. 3.

Nervous system
Acute intoxication; 'black-outs'
Persistent brain damage:
   Wernicke's encephalopathy
   Korsakoff's syndrome
   cerebellar degeneration
   dementia
Cerebrovascular disease:
   strokes, especially in young
   people
   subarachnoid haemorrhage
   subdural haematoma after head
   injury
Withdrawal symptoms:
   tremor, hallucinations, fits
Nerve and muscle damage:
   weakness, paralysis, burning
   sensations in hands and feet

Liver
Infiltration of liver with fat
Alcoholic hepatitis
Cirrhosis and eventual liver failure
Liver cancer

Gastrointestinal system
Reflux of acid into the oesophagus
Tearing and occasionally rupture of
   the oesophagus
Cancer of the oesophagus
Gastritis
Aggravation and impaired healing
   of peptic ulcers
Diarrhoea and impaired absorption
   of food
Chronic inflammation of the
   pancreas leading in some to
   diabetes and malabsorption of
   food

Nutrition
Malnutrition from reduced intake of
   food, toxic effects of alcohol on
   intestine, and impaired
   metabolism, leading to weight
   loss
Obesity, particularly in early stages
   of heavy drinking

Heart and circulatory system
Abnormal rhythms
High blood pressure
Chronic heart muscle damage
   leading to heart failure

Respiratory system
Fractured ribs
Pneumonia from inhalation of
   vomit

Endocrine system
Overproduction of cortisol leading
   to obesity, acne, increased facial
   hair, and high blood pressure
Condition mimicking over-activity
   of the thyroid with loss of weight,
   anxiety, palpitations, sweating,
   and tremor
Severe fall in blood sugar,
   sometimes leading to coma
Intense facial flushing in many
   diabetics taking the anti-diabetic
   drug chlorpropamide

Reproductive system
In men, loss of libido, reduced
   potency, shrinkage in size of
   testes and penis, reduced or
   absent sperm formation and so
   infertility, and loss of sexual
   hair
In women, sexual difficulties,
   menstrual irregularities, and
   shrinkage of breasts and external
   genitalia

Occupation and accidents
Impaired work performance and
   decision making
Increased risk and severity of
   accidents

The fetus, the child, and the family
Damage to the fetus and the fetal
   alcohol syndrome
Acute intoxication in young
   children:
   hypothermia, low blood sugar
   levels, depressed respiration
Effect on physical development and
   behaviour of the child through
   heavy drinking by parents

Interaction of alcohol with medicinal substances
Increased likelihood of unwanted
   effects of drugs
Reduced effectiveness of medicines

Table 3.2 United Kingdom alcohol consumption per head of population and convictions for public drunkenness, drinking and driving convictions, cirrhosis mortality and hospital admissions for alcohol dependence, 1970–84. *Source:* Ref. 4.

Year	UK alcohol consumption per head in litres of pure alcohol	UK drunkenness convictions per 10,000 pop.	Drinking and driving convictions in Britain per 10,000 pop.	Cirrhosis deaths in England and Wales per 100,000 pop.	English hospital first admissions for alcohol dependence per 100,000 pop.
1970	7.03	22.3	8.4	3.71	5.17
1971	7.37	23.4	11.7	4.19	5.70
1972	7.79	24.1	13.8	4.41	6.19
1973	8.61	26.6	16.0	4.77	7.34
1974	8.85	27.7	16.3	4.63	8.11
1975	8.82	27.9	16.6	4.82	8.40
1976	9.28	28.6	14.1	4.94	8.68
1977	8.81	28.2	12.7	4.73	9.17
1978	9.50	27.5	14.1	4.97	9.13
1979	9.79	29.9	15.6	5.60	9.74
1980	9.33	30.9	18.2	5.64	10.96
1981	8.89	27.1	16.5	5.59	10.55
1982	8.67	26.1	17.0	5.42	8.91
1983	8.83	25.7[a]	22.3[b]	5.47	8.63
1984	9.21	22.1[a]	22.8	5.67	9.46

Note: All figures refer to the population aged fifteen or over.
a These figures are for England and Wales only.
b The 1981 Road Transport Act introduced evidential breath-testing machines in May 1983.

Recommended limits of alcohol consumption

The usual assessment of alcohol intake is in units. The number of units per measure of drink, and the suggested limits of consumption are set out below:

Units of alcohol and recommended limits

One unit (= 8g alcohol) is equivalent to:

  half a pint of beer
  one small glass of sherry
  one small glass of wine
  one single (English) measure of spirits

Such assessments are approximate because of the varying alcoholic content of different wines (8–14%) and beers (3–8%).

- A suggested guide for **low risk drinking** is up to:

      21 units a week for men
      14 units a week for women
      with preferably some drink-free days

- It is **dangerous** to drink persistently more than:

      50 units a week for men
      35 units a week for women

Such advice can only be a guideline because of the wide individual variation in reactions to this drug, but the upper limits indicate an overall significantly increased risk of one of the alcohol-induced disturbances described above.

Alcohol metabolism in men and women

The difference between alcohol metabolism in men and women is based on two pieces of evidence.[20] In pre-menopausal women after a standard dose of alcohol per kg body weight the blood pressure rose higher than in men. Women have a lower level than men of the alcohol destroying enzyme gastric alcohol dehydrogenase, leading to higher blood levels of alcohol.[21] The higher levels may also be related to the smaller proportion of water in the body mass of younger women (50%) compared with men (60%) and post-menopausal women. Furthermore, Wilkinson *et al.*[22] found that women alcoholics were more predisposed to develop

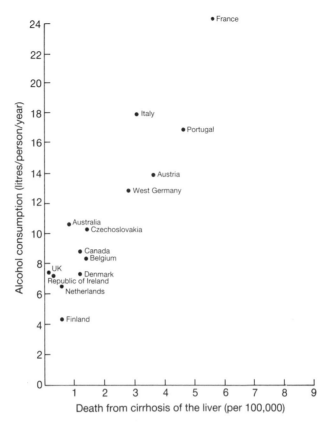

Fig. 3.1 *Comparison of alcohol consumption and deaths from cirrhosis of the liver in 12 countries.* Source: *Popham RE et al. 1975.*[19]

liver disease than men, while Williams and Davis[23] found a higher proportion of severe liver disease in pre-menopausal women, although their alcohol intake was less; this difference was not found in post-menopausal women. Whether the difference in the metabolism of alcohol described in young women accounts for the different patterns of liver disease is as yet unknown. Such differences between men and women have not been demonstrated for other types of alcohol-induced physical damage but the search has been less thorough.

Strategies for prevention

The three potential strategies for prevention are:

1. Health education
2. Screening, and
3. Legislation.

Health education

Education about alcohol faces a difficult challenge.[24] The drinking habit is widely enjoyed and general advice to cut down consumption is met with ambivalence and disbelief by many. Some educators now feel that expensive broad-based education programmes have little to offer[15] and believe that greater chance of success will be achieved by concentrating on vulnerable subjects and where drinking could cause dangerous situations. Examples are: pregnant women, children, teenagers, drivers and the work place. The number and variety of both government and voluntary agents who could potentially be engaged in activities to educate about alcohol consumption is large but poorly co-ordinated—there are at least fifteen government departments with some responsibility for this problem. Ideally, these activities should be co-ordinated, and there are now some encouraging examples of co-ordinated action at local level.[7]

Screening and case finding

Screening for alcohol misuse can be undertaken by a doctor when carrying out a general health check on an apparently healthy person, or when a patient presents with a specific complaint. A drinking history should be taken as routinely as a smoking history (see Chapter 2). Patients should be asked how much they drink; if vague, they should be asked what they drank last week and whether they drink every day. It can often be helpful for the doctor to suggest an amount and then negotiate; for example, if the patient says he takes a whisky in the evening ask if it is home poured without a measure, and if so suggest it is a triple because no one can taste a single! The amount may then be converted into units and the patient told about the guidelines on what are considered safe amounts of alcohol.

Patients presenting with disorders such as hypertension and depression should always be asked about alcohol consumption as such disorders may be associated with an alcohol problem. Blood tests can be helpful and are often found to be abnormal during a routine test or when the patient is investigated for intercurrent disease, the doctor often being unaware that the patient has an alcohol problem. The MCV is frequently raised; alcohol abuse is probably the commonest cause of macrocytosis in Great Britain today.

Gamma GT, an enzyme derived from the liver, is raised in up to 50% of people who are heavy drinkers. However, the distribution curve of the normal range is skew and many normal people have a level above the so-called upper normal limit of 40 units per litre. Analysis of many

thousands of sera from subjects screened at a private clinic showed that
the upper level of 95% of the population is 80 units/litre and that by
no means all of those with levels above this figure abused alcohol. Body
weight was an independent variable that influenced the gamma GT
concentration. In addition, other microsomal inducing drugs, such as
phenytoin, increase the concentration of this enzyme in the blood, and
of course so do co-existent non-alcoholic biliary tract and liver disease.
Raised gamma GT levels due to alcohol misuse will decrease with
abstinence from alcohol, and this test can then act as a useful monitor
of the success of counselling.

Case identification, when the effects of alcohol become overt, can be
undertaken by teachers who are involved in investigating a change of
a child's behaviour, social workers helping a disturbed family and
personnel officers at the work place who are becoming aware that poor
performance may be due to a drinking problem.

Legislation

Changing the price is the most effective way to change the overall
consumption of alcohol in a country, and thus alcohol-related death
and illness in the population. Many studies in different countries have
confirmed this. The real price of alcohol in Great Britain fell between
1950 and 1980; *pari passu* there was a rise in consumption and a rise in
deaths from cirrhosis. In Denmark, there was a clear correlation

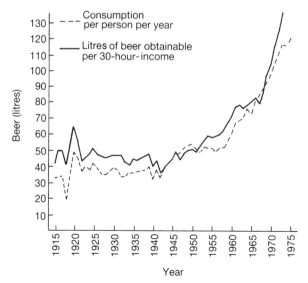

Fig. 3.2 *Relationship between price of beer and consumer purchasing, Denmark 1915–75. Source: Neilson and Sorensen, 1979.*[25]

between consumption of beer per head and purchasing power—expressed as the number of litres of beer obtainable for thirty hours' work.[25] Currently, the British government seems to be ambivalent about raising price as a method of control. As pointed out earlier in this chapter, in 1983 the drink industry generated £6,000 million and 250,000 jobs, so industrial and Treasury pressures may be exerted against this method of control. Furthermore, price increases are unpopular with the public and increase inflation because the cost of alcohol, like tobacco, is included in the Retail Price Index (see Appendix).

Suggestions that advertising should be limited and should carry health warnings, as for tobacco, have not been agreed. The industry spends over £150 million a year on advertising, claiming that its purpose is merely to persuade consumers to change to or to remain with the advertised brand and not to increase consumption. The validity of the argument and the potential harm in persuading the public that drinking is desirable and glamorous, have been much disputed but no conclusive data are available.

Drunken driving was initially reduced by the introduction of the breathalyzer but the effect has levelled off. There has been pressure for use of different variations of 'random breathalyzing' and more stringent limits for alcohol levels above which cars may not be driven but so far without success. It is strongly suggested that one of the many government agencies engaged on work to prevent alcohol abuse is placed in overall charge and a more co-ordinated government effort undertaken.

RECOMMENDATIONS

1   The price of alcohol should be increased at least in line with inflation or to the average amount of working time needed to earn the cost of a bottle of spirits. The pros and cons of more stringent measures of price control should be considered, for example, exclusion of alcohol—and tobacco—from the RPI.

2   Advertisement of alcohol should be curtailed.

3   The alcohol contents in units and grams should be stated clearly on all containers of alcoholic drinks, and they should carry a health warning.

4   The use of low alcohol beer, lager and wine should be encouraged as an alternative to the beverages of standard and high alcohol content.

5 Medical practitioners should be aware of the protean manifestations of alcohol abuse and should take a history of the drinking habits of all patients. Patients should be advised about safe drinking limits.

6 Health education about alcohol should be targeted at:

- professions responsible for the wellbeing of others, such as health care workers, teachers and personnel officers, so that they can recognise and, if possible, counsel and know to whom to refer, people who are thought to be drinking to excess.

- vulnerable subjects, such as children, teenagers, pregnant women, drivers, and those at risk by virtue of their occupation.

7 The large number of government agencies and departments with responsibility for alcohol policy should be better co-ordinated.

4 Healthy diets

The burden of nutrition related disease

The relationship of diet to health has long been known—Hippocrates first wrote of the relationship between food and health in 400 BC. Although essential to life, food can produce health problems in man because of malnutrition, overnutrition or the necessity of achieving an appropriate balance of all the necessary nutrients. In the UK in the 1990s undernutrition is rare, although in some sections of the community lack of education or poverty are the reasons for inappropriate diets. However, as in other countries of the developed world, a more widespread problem is that of overnutrition and its consequent health effects.

The medical conditions most frequently associated with nutrition usually have several causes. However, diet plays a large part in the burden of deaths from circulatory disorders and cancers[1] as well as in deaths due to disorders of the digestive system, and metabolic diseases. Together, these disease categories are an important component of mortality in England and Wales.[2] Moreover, in the past 40 years diet-related disease has had an increasing impact on total mortality.

Overnutrition and obesity

The most obvious effect of overeating, defined here as the consumption of more calories than are warranted for activity level or energy expenditure, is obesity which, when severe, is associated with numerous health and social problems including coronary heart disease, cerebrovascular disease, type 2 (non-insulin dependent) diabetes, gall stones, respiratory disorders, arthritis, hypertension, and cancer of the gallbladder and endometrium. Obesity can be a chronically persistent problem, with the overweight child or young adult more likely to remain overweight in adulthood,[3] although most overweight adults were not overweight in childhood.

What is obesity?

So what is 'obesity'? A popular method of establishing whether and to what extent a patient is obese is the use of the *Body Mass Index (BMI)*. This was accepted as an appropriate method of classifying body weight by the First International Conference on Body Weight Control.[4]

BMI is a formula[5] (weight in kg divided by (height in m)^2) which classifies:

- optimum body weight — BMI of 20–24.9;
- overweight (also known as grade 1 obesity) — BMI 25-29.9;
- classical or grade 2 obesity — BMI 30–39.9, and
- grade 3 obesity — BMI of 40 or more.

Many European studies employ the Broca index which essentially gives the same answers. These measures can give the physician an indicator of inappropriate weight for an individual's height, but can only ever act as a guide, since no distinction is drawn between fat and lean tissue.

The extent of the obesity problem

Public health activity has great potential to reduce or prevent obesity. In Great Britain in 1984, 36 per cent of the adult population were either overweight, or obese to some extent (see Table 4.1). By 1987 this had risen to 40%. Between 1980 and 1987 the proportion of adults with a BMI of over 30 rose from 7% to 10%.[6] In the UK, the prevalence of obesity increases with age for both men and women, rising steadily for women (ie the proportion of women with BMI of 30–40 increases steadily between ages 20 and 60 years), but more sharply after age 35 years in men.[7]

Reduction of obesity

Obesity is caused by consuming too many calories for the energy levels expended. Energy dense diets are often high in fat, which is a concentrated source of calories, and foods high in fat are often also high in sugar.

Table 4.1 Weight categories, Great Britain 1984

Body Mass Index (BMI)	Percent of population
<20	12
20–24	53
25–29	28
30–34	6
>34	2

Source: Knight I, 1989[8]

High intakes of alcohol can also contribute to obesity. Guidelines to aid weight reduction generally include restrictions in fat, sugar and alcohol consumption, a smaller reduction in the intake of starchy foods and animal proteins, and encouragement to increase the wholegrain cereal content of the diet and to eat more fruit and vegetables. Calorie reduced diets may potentially contain inadequate amounts of vitamins and minerals if the foods chosen are not varied, and for this reason 'fad' diets that provide a very restricted variety of foodstuffs should not be encouraged. An increase in energy expenditure during attempted weight loss is also encouraged. There is also some evidence for the suggestion that feeding patterns (ie frequency and timing of meals) may have some influence on weight although the evidence is by no means conclusive.[9]

Healthy diets

There is more than just optimum weight maintenance to making a diet healthy. The balance of different foodstuffs is also important.

Fats

Current recommendations for adults suggest that the percentage energy contribution from fats should be reduced to a maximum of 33% of total energy intake, not including alcohol, with only 10% being saturated fats.[6] The Committee on Medical Aspects of Food Policy (COMA) recommendations for the UK are broadly in keeping with those of James[10] (Table 4.2), although COMA makes no specific recommendations for protein intake, as this is rarely a problem in the UK, whereas the James (1988) recommendations are intended to be applied internationally. In 1984, COMA recommended an average daily intake of total fat of 77–87 g per day (or 31–35% of energy), with a recommended polyunsaturated/saturated ratio of 0.45.[11] They recommended a saturated fatty acid intake of 37 g (or 15% of energy), and an unsaturated fatty acid intake of 8.6–16.7 g per day (or 3.5–6.8% of energy). In the UK the total energy derived from fat has increased substantially, from 36.8% of the total food energy in 1950, to 42.6% in 1982.[11] Since then, total calories, including fat, have come down but the proportion of energy derived from fat has remained stable, being around 42% in 1988. The recommended reduction is aimed at substantially reducing both mortality and morbidity from cardiovascular disease and a number of other conditions already mentioned. It should be noted that these recommendations are not intended for infants or children under the age

Table 4.2 Intermediate and ultimate nutritional goals for the general population of Europe

Dietary constituent	Intermediate goal	Ultimate goal
Percentage of total energy derived from		
– Carbohydrate	>40%	45–55%
– Protein	12–13%	12–13%
– Sugar	10%	10%
– Total fat	35%	20–30%
– Saturated fat	15%	10%
Polyunsaturated/saturated fatty acid ratio	>0.5	>1.0
Cholesterol (mg/4.18 mJ)	–	<100
Salt (g/day)	7–8	5
Fibre (g/day)	30	>30

Source: James 1988[10]

of five who normally take a large proportion of their energy intake from cows' milk.[6]

Cholesterol and fatty acids

The mean plasma cholesterol levels of healthy adults vary widely between countries, for example from 3.0 mmol/l in Bushmen and Masai, to greater than 7.0 mmol/l in eastern Finland. No other common plasma variable shows similarly wide variation. Only in countries in which average plasma cholesterol exceeds 5.2 mmol/l (as in Britain) is coronary heart disease common. In the UK over half of all men and women in the 25–59 year age group have plasma cholesterol levels in excess of 5.5 mmol/l.[12]

Raised plasma cholesterol levels are a major risk factor for coronary heart disease. It has been said that a 1% reduction in plasma cholesterol concentration in middle-aged men should result in a reduction of 2% in the incidence of coronary heart disease.[13]

Total plasma cholesterol can be subdivided into low density and high density lipoproteins. Low density lipoproteins are thought to be harmful, whereas high density lipoproteins (HDL) are thought to exert some protective influence against coronary heart disease. The evidence is not yet so strong that reductions in low density lipoproteins are being universally recommended, but there is a definite trend towards encouraging the consumption of foods such as fish which may increase high density lipoprotein levels, although there may also be other mechanisms whereby they protect against coronary heart disease.

The main determinants of total and low density lipoprotein (LDL) cholesterol levels in plasma are dietary lipids (fats). It is generally accepted that a reduction in the intake of calories from fat in the diet will reduce levels of plasma total and LDL cholesterol.[14] When such reduction is achieved in conjunction with an increase in the ratio of polyunsaturated fatty acids to saturated fatty acids (the P/S ratio) a greater reduction in levels of these plasma lipids has been observed.[14] Several European studies have demonstrated an association between the balance of fatty acid consumed in the habitual diet (ie balance of saturated or unsaturated) and later evidence of coronary heart disease.[15,16] There is still controversy as to whether changes in dietary cholesterol itself in a habitual diet can have a significant influence on its concentration in the plasma.

Current research is being undertaken to investigate the hypothesis that water soluble fibre (eg from foods such as oats, beans, peas and legumes) exerts some protective influence against coronary heart disease—possibly by reducing cholesterol levels. Fruit and vegetable fibre may also reduce plasma cholesterol levels. Another current research issue is the role of free radicals,* agents which can destabilise fatty acids and hence may have a pathogenic role in coronary heart disease.

The progression of coronary heart disease, once it is established, may also be influenced by plasma cholesterol levels;—there is evidence indicating that low plasma cholesterol levels may have some influence in retarding the progress of the disease. The role of plasma cholesterol in the development of heart disease is also discussed in Chapter 5.

Salt

The WHO Expert Committee on Prevention of Coronary Heart Disease has suggested that a reduction in the consumption of salt among hypertensive individuals may reduce the burden of cardiovascular disease since excessive salt consumption may be linked with hypertension

---

*When oxygen is incompletely utilised for electron transfer superoxide radical and other oxygen species are formed which are highly reactive and generate a chain of other reactive radicals which can damage important molecules. Free radicals are important in reperfusion injury and are thought to play a role in the pathogenesis of several important diseases, including coronary atheroma.

which is a major risk factor for both coronary heart disease and cerebrovascular disease.[17,18] While it is known that salt reduction leads to a fall in blood pressure in hypertensive patients, its preventive effect in normotensive individuals is not yet proven.[6] However, a recent overview of many international and within-country observational studies of salt consumption and blood pressure levels, and of 78 trials of salt reduction, has concluded that the effect of salt on blood pressure has been underestimated in the past, and that sustained moderate salt reduction lowers blood pressure in normotensive as well as hypertensive individuals.[19] The role of salt in the development of hypertension and subsequently of coronary heart disease and cerebrovascular disease is also mentioned in Chapter 5.

Since UK average salt consumption (around 10–12 g/day per person) is more than is physiologically required, an overall recommendation that consumption be reduced can be made. It is recommended by WHO that no more than 5 g salt per day should be consumed[10] and that fewer highly processed foods should be eaten because of their high salt content. It is accepted that this may be an unrealistic target which would require major changes not only in household food preparation but also in manufacturing and therefore an interim aim of a reduction, to 7–8 g of salt per day, has been suggested.

In addition to the influence of salt consumption on hypertension, the regular consumption of salty or pickled foods and cured meats has also been associated with gastric cancer (see Chapter 6).

Adequate potassium and magnesium in the diet may also help to control blood pressure.

Dietary fibre

Dietary fibre is a term used to describe a varying group of plant food elements that are resistant to human digestive enzymes. Their main component is non-starch polysaccharides which are complex carbo-hydrates. World Health Organisation (WHO) guidelines recommend a total dietary fibre consumption level in excess of 30 g per day, and COMA recently proposed that the average consumption in the UK should be of the order of 18 g per day.[6] Currently, in the UK, average consumption of non-starch polysaccharides is 11–13 g per day of which about half comes from vegetables and 40% from cereals.[6]

Increasing consumption of cereals, whole grains, roots, fruit and vegetables denotes an increase in dietary fibre consumption which has a number of direct effects on health—for example, prevention of constipa-tion and possibly of diverticular disease. Dietary fibre is also increasingly

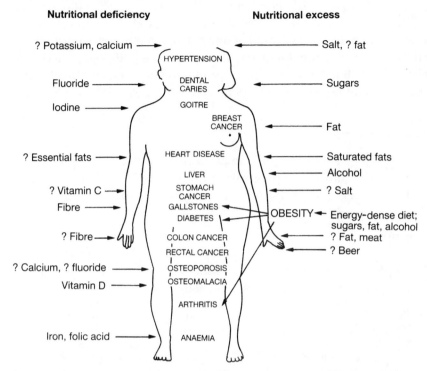

Nutritional deficiency   **Nutritional excess**

? Potassium, calcium ⟶   HYPERTENSION   ⟵ Salt, ? fat

Fluoride ⟶   DENTAL CARIES   ⟵ Sugars

Iodine ⟶   GOITRE

BREAST CANCER   ⟵ Fat

? Essential fats ⟶   HEART DISEASE   ⟵ Saturated fats

LIVER   ⟵ Alcohol

? Vitamin C ⟶   STOMACH CANCER   ⟵ ? Salt

Fibre ⟶   GALLSTONES
         DIABETES   OBESITY ⟵ Energy-dense diet; sugars, fat, alcohol

? Fibre ⟶   COLON CANCER   ⟵ ? Fat, meat
            RECTAL CANCER   ⟵ ? Beer

? Calcium, ? fluoride ⟶   OSTEOPOROSIS

Vitamin D ⟶   OSTEOMALACIA

ARTHRITIS

Iron, folic acid ⟶   ANAEMIA

Fig. 4.1 *Health problems in Europe and their possible association with diet.* Note: *Individual susceptibility to the prevailing diet is important in both nutritional deficiency and excess. The nutritional components have only been tentatively linked to many of the conditions shown.* Source: *James (1988)*[10].

linked with a number of other conditions (Fig. 4.1). It has been suggested that patients whose diets do not include adequate fruit and green vegetables are more prone to various cancers of the digestive tract. Enthusiasm for the hypothesis that linked a lack of dietary fibre itself and large bowel cancer has waned somewhat, and it has been suggested that any food which reaches the large bowel and acts as a substrate for bacteria would have a similar influence. Research into this issue must continue. There is also an ongoing debate about the hypothesis that water-soluble dietary fibre may lower plasma cholesterol levels.[20]

Complex carbohydrate

Complex carbohydrates (for example bread, potatoes, pasta, rice) provide a good energy source which is essential in a diet with reduced fat and sugar.

Simple sugar

Reduction in the consumption of simple sugar has an important impact on the incidence of dental caries. Taking less sugar also helps to control obesity. It has recently been proposed that non-milk extrinsic sugars should not exceed 60 g per day or 10% of total dietary energy.[6]

Vitamins and minerals

A healthy diet should contain an appropriate balance of vitamins and minerals, in addition to progressing toward the WHO's intermediate and ultimate goals for all the major nutrient groups.

Vitamins

Examples of essential vitamins, of which deficiency or excess can have serious implications, include the following:

- *Vitamin A* occurs in liver and in green and yellow vegetables. Deficiency leads to night blindness and skin disorders, and excess consumption over a prolonged period may be toxic, especially in pregnancy. Recent advice from the Chief Medical Officer is for pregnant women to avoid excessive consumption of liver, previously recommended because of its iron content, because of the possible toxic effects of excess vitamin A on the fetus.

- *Vitamin B1* (thiamin) occurs in many foods and by UK regulation white flour must contain a minimum amount. Deficiency of thiamin in a diet rich in carbohydrate or alcohol leads to beri-beri and Wernicke's encephalopathy.[21]

- *Vitamin B12* occurs in animal products and fortified breakfast cereals. Deficiency leads to macrocytic anaemia and nerve cell degeneration.[21] However deficiency most frequently occurs as a result of an inability to utilise that which is available, due to deficiency of some co-factor.

- *Folic acid*, found in leafy green vegetables, prevents anaemia. There has been a suggestion that folic acid deficiency in women leads to neural tube defects in the fetus,[22] and it has now been shown that administration of folic acid to women who have had a previous neural tube defect fetus reduces the risk of a subsequent pregnancy being similarly affected.[23]

- *Vitamin C* (ascorbic acid) occurs in vegetables and fruit and promotes iron absorption. Deficiency leads to bleeding gums and scurvy. There is little scientific basis for the claim that it prevents the common cold. There is increasing interest in the hypothesis that vitamin C may exert some preventive influence in the development of cardiovascular disease and cancer of the stomach.

- *Vitamin D* occurs in milk products and fortified margarine, and is synthesised in the body under the influence of sunlight. It maintains blood calcium levels and deficiency leads to rickets in children, particularly those that are kept indoors for long periods. Deficiency has also been associated with osteomalacia in adults. Asian populations living in Britain, and the elderly, are at risk of vitamin D deficiency. Excess vitamin D can be toxic especially in infants.

- *Vitamin E* which occurs in vegetable oils, is thought to protect against coronary heart disease. Its role is now being tested in a large-scale controlled trial.

Vitamins in relation to cancer prevention are discussed in Chapter 6.

Minerals

- *Iron*. About 20% of iron in the British diet comes from meat,[21] the remainder from cereals and root vegetables. Inadequate iron intake leads to anaemia.

- *Calcium* occurs in milk and cheese, and is added to bread; skimmed milk contains as much calcium as full-fat milk. Adequate calcium intake is thought to be important in early life and during the adolescent growth spurt for preventing osteoporosis in women in later life (see Chapter 11).

- *Iodine* prevents goitre, but deficiency is rare in the UK since iodine added to cattle feed reaches humans through milk.

- *Zinc* is essential for growth and healing. The best sources are meat and dairy products. Zinc is poorly absorbed from the gut, particularly when diets are rich in cereals and dietary fibre. Zinc deficiency may result in stunting; vegetarians should therefore be made aware of the risk of deficiency.[21]

- *Aluminium* The possible damaging effects of exposure to aluminium in drinking water has aroused much recent interest, but the doses received are likely to be trivial compared with those from medicinal sources.

- *Fluoride* is important in the prevention of dental caries.[24]

People with special needs

The guidelines given above are necessarily very general and do not take account of the numerous groups of people with special needs—for example, the elderly, the young, pregnant women and people choosing to follow particular dietary regimes.

The elderly

In the UK, the elderly are a population group potentially at risk of nutritional deficiency. One survey found that of 365 elderly people living in their own houses, 7% were diagnosed as clinically under-nourished.[25] Dietary recommendations are currently the same as for any adult, but it has been suggested that their particular needs for nutrients may be greater due to less efficient absorption. Diet in the elderly is discussed in Chapter 11.

Children and adolescents

Babies should be breast-fed where possible. The diet of the small child is important from the point of view that taste preferences are established at this time, and appropriate health education of parents can help establish healthier eating patterns from infancy onwards.

Obviously children and adolescents should receive enough food while they are growing rapidly. Calcium intake, which is important for the development of bones during the growth spurt, should also be adequate.

Pregnant and lactating women

Advice on optimum levels of weight gain during pregnancy should always be given. Iron supplements are advisable for pregnant women with low haemoglobin levels (eg below 10.5 g/100 ml). Increased consumption of fibre may protect against the risk of developing haemorrhoids although the precise aetiology of haemorrhoids in pregnancy is unclear. Folic acid but not multi-vitamin supplements protects against neural tube defects, at least in women who have had a previous affected pregnancy. Pregnant women should limit their consumption of alcohol (see Chapter 3). Pregnant women should be advised to avoid unpasteurised soft cheeses (see Food Safety below).

Vegetarians/vegans

Lacto-ovo-vegetarians (the most commonly occurring) are only rarely at risk of dietary deficiency if they eat a mixed and varied diet. But vegans can be at risk of vitamin B12 deficiency and calcium deficiency. Vitamin B12 supplements in vegans are recommended during pregnancy and lactation, since there is some evidence of neurological damage, and of rickets due to vitamin D deficiency, in breast fed babies of vegan mothers.[22]

Food safety

Reports about lack of food hygiene have often been linked to food preparation in institutionalised settings, such as in the Stanley Royd

Hospital food poisoning outbreak in 1984, but have not aroused much general concern.

Infective agents

Recent media publicity in the UK about infective agents in the general food supply have caused much greater concern and had a greater impact. In 1989, the media reported possible widespread presence of salmonella in eggs, and a short-term but devastating impact on the egg industry followed. To a lesser extent the same thing happened with later publicity about listeria in soft cheeses and bovine spongiform encephalopathy (BSE) in beef. The risks to the general public from these food contaminants are hard to quantify but are probably very small. However the risk to the fetus of listeria infection is sufficient to warrant advice to pregnant women to avoid unpasteurised soft cheeses.

Hygiene

Since the majority of incidents of food poisoning occur as a result of food contamination in the home, it is essential that education in food hygiene and safe food handling is adequate (see Chapter 8). The major role of the physician on food safety is in giving advice regarding appropriate shopping, preparation and storage of food. The use of refrigerator thermometers should be encouraged and people should be aware that food should be stored in the refrigerator between 0 and 4°C.

Additives

Food additives have also roused increased concern—it is postulated that they may be associated with hyperactivity, lethargy, appetite and sleeping problems in children. There has been no conclusive epidemiological evidence to back up this assertion, but there is a need for continuous monitoring. Co-factors may influence a child's sensitivity to food additives, for example allergy, intolerance or reactivity to other naturally occurring foodstuffs such as dairy produce. The physician may be able to help the parent of the child with food allergies — the best approach often being a temporary restriction of foods suspected of causing allergies. It should be noted that genuine food allergy is very rare.[26,27] Restriction of natural foods such as dairy produce or wheat products needs careful monitoring by a dietitian if allergy to these is suspected.

Preservation methods

Current trends against the widespread use of chemical preservatives in food have been widely applauded. However this presents nutritionists with the new problem of how to keep food fresh, without additives and without severely damaging the nutritional content of the food. Food irradiation is currently under scrutiny, but the Department of Health is satisfied that nutritional losses from irradiated food are not great, and that irradiation at the specified level does not pose any risk to human health.[28] Food irradiation at the specified level became legal in the UK in January 1991.

Surveillance

Dangers from food additives and irradiation are probably greatly outweighed by the risks of infection which they help to prevent. These issues of food safety outlined above, highlight the need for constant, high-quality surveillance of food standards. The medical profession has an important role in keeping this on the political agenda.

Progress in the UK toward a healthy diet

Dietary habits are changing in the UK. Despite the often conflicting advice meted out to them via the media and sometimes the medical profession, the British public are fundamentally changing the contents of their shopping baskets (see Table 4.3).

The trends are encouraging, with consumption of red meat and dairy produce declining, with butter largely replaced by other forms of fat, increasing consumption of fruit and fruit products and a huge decline in consumption of white bread and increased consumption of brown and wholemeal bread. UK total home consumption of fat has slightly declined over time, and the balance of saturated to unsaturated fat has changed in favour of a higher P/S ratio[29] (Fig. 4.2). However, there is some evidence that people tend to eat out increasingly frequently; the meals they eat may not necessarily exhibit the same encouraging tendencies as the food they buy to prepare at home.

The doctor's role in promoting healthy diets

The general practitioner and the primary care team have an essential role to play in monitoring weight and nutritional status in their patients, advising and treating those with obesity and referring them to dietitians or self-help groups as appropriate. The lack of fully trained

Table 4.3   Trends in average quantities of selected foods purchased each week for home consumption in Great Britain, 1961 to 1987 (1980 = 100%)

Type of Food	Year			
	1961	1971	1981	1987
Dairy produce	106	109	99	90
Meat	103	97	90	73
Poultry	36	73	109	119
Fish/fish products	119	107	103	106
Butter	153	137	91	53
Margarine/all other fats	81	84	102	110
Fresh vegetables	119	109	100	93
Other vegetables/vegetable products	61	78	105	120
Fresh fruit	83	96	96	97
Other fruit/fruit products	88	92	109	148
White bread	165	137	100	73
Brown/wholemeal bread	58	55	100	151
Sugar	162	141	99	67

Source: Adapted from Table 7.11 *Purchases of selected foods for home consumption*. Central Statistical Office.[30]

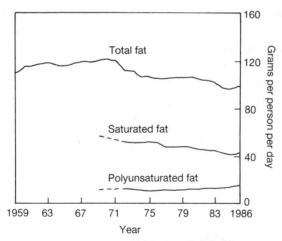

Fig. 4.2 *Fat and fatty acid content of the average British diet.* Source: *Central Statistical Office.*[29]

specialist dietitians in the NHS places more responsibility on the role of the doctor as an adviser on diet. It is now a requirement of the GP contract to discuss life-style with patients, particularly eating habits, and to weigh patients regularly.

The role of the doctor in prevention of morbidity associated with diet was demonstrated particularly effectively in the North Karelia community project in Finland in the early 1980s, in which practitioners were said to have provided a valuable source of information, advice and leadership in the project which had a significant impact (at least in the short term) on risk factors for coronary heart disease. In the UK, the 'Look After Your Heart' campaign of the Health Education Council (now Health Education Authority) had some impact on increasing awareness of risk factors for coronary heart disease, especially among the lower paid sections of the community at whom it was targeted— a group who are normally least affected by life-style messages. This campaign showed that the doctor could have a vital role in encouraging community initiatives, workplace initiatives and local projects aimed at increasing awareness of heart disease.

Government's role in promoting healthy diets

Governments have a far reaching role in the promotion of healthy diets, for example in legislation about the fat content of meat and processed food, food labelling, publication of recommended dietary guidelines, legislation about the addition of salt to food, addition of fluoride to water supplies, the standards of institutional food, and the employment (in local government) of environmental health officers. Agricultural subsidies have an effect on the national diet and could be used to influence it beneficially. The medical profession has a role to play in advising governments on these issues, and in ensuring that governments are kept informed of new developments, and of the views of the profession toward education policy, pricing policies and policies toward advertising, so that the public are aware of what constitutes a healthy diet and that it is available to them.

RECOMMENDATIONS

1   People should be advised to:

- reduce consumption of *fat* (particularly saturated fat);
- avoid fatty foods such as processed meats;
- replace some red meat in the diet with fish or poultry;
- use cooking methods that do not add fat;

- reduce the consumption of full fat dairy products and replace them with lower fat alternatives;
- substitute polyunsaturated fats (eg soft margarine and vegetable oils) for saturated fats (eg butter, hard margarine, lard, dripping); and
- avoid fatty snacks such as nuts, crisps, biscuits, etc.

2   Plasma *cholesterol* levels can be lowered by reducing total dietary fat and increasing the polyunsaturated fatty acids to saturated fatty acids ratio (P/S ratio). Increased vegetable and fruit fibre consumption may also help reduce plasma cholesterol levels. The addition of water soluble fibre to the diet may also have an impact on plasma cholesterol levels, although the evidence on this is not conclusive.

3   The proportion of total energy intake in the diet derived from *starchy carbohydrate*, such as bread, pasta and rice, should be increased to provide an adequate energy supply in a reduced fat and sugar diet. Consumption of sugar and confectionery should be reduced.

4   A raised intake of dietary fibre should be achieved by increasing the consumption of whole grains, cereals, fruits and vegetables and by eating wholemeal bread rather than white.

5   Little or no salt should be added in cooking or at the table and salty food should be avoided.

6   Industry should be encouraged to reduce the fat and salt content of processed food, and where possible food should be labelled to show its constituents.

7   Home economics courses in schools should include education about healthy diets, and school meals should conform with the above recommendations.

8   Hospitals and other institutions should likewise provide healthy diets.

5 Heart disease and stroke

In 1989, diseases of the circulatory system were responsible for 264,600 (46%) of the 576,872 deaths in England and Wales. Of these, 67,692 (12% of the total) were attributed to cerebrovascular disease; most of the remaining deaths were due to coronary heart disease. In the UK some 100,000 individuals experience their first stroke every year and some 300,000 suffer an acute myocardial infarction.

Congenital heart disease (which affects some 4,000–5,000 children born each year) and rheumatic and valvular heart disease, although relatively uncommon, are important because of the young age of the individuals who suffer from them and because of the frequent need for highly skilled surgery in their treatment.

Coronary heart disease

Pathology

Coronary heart disease can be regarded as having two phases, although this is a considerable over-simplification. The first is a gradual build-up of atheromatous material in plaques in the walls of the coronary arteries; this is initially asymptomatic but may lead to angina. Secondly, the plaques may rupture and thrombosis become superimposed; this phenomenon is the usual basis for the acute syndromes of unstable angina and myocardial infarction.

The size of the problem

In England and Wales, coronary heart disease is the commonest cause of death in males in every decade from 35 upwards; in women it is second only to cancer. In 1989, 18,476 men and 5,194 women under the age of 65 died from this cause.[1] Of the 1,065,000 life years lost by men dying before the age of 65, almost half (532,000) were attributed to heart disease[2] (see also Fig. 1.2).

Precise information on the prevalence of angina is not available, but coronary heart disease is probably the most important single cause of prolonged absence from work and has immense economic implications both because of loss of productive capacity and because of the high costs of treatment. In 1986/87 in Great Britain, diseases of the circulatory system accounted for 68 million of the 266 million days of certified incapacity in men.

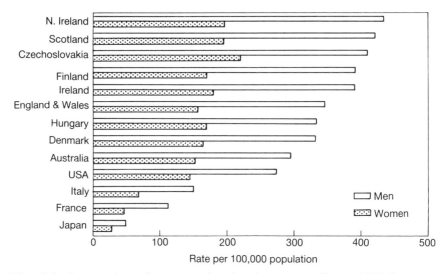

Fig. 5.1 *Coronary heart disease rate for selected countries; all ages 1986.* Source: *Coronary Prevention Group/British Heart Foundation (1988)* Statistical information on coronary heart disease.

There are great variations in the mortality from coronary heart disease in different countries (Fig. 5.1). Striking reductions in coronary mortality have occurred in the USA, Canada and Australia; these have been paralleled by comparable reductions in overall mortality, making it unlikely that these reductions are artifactual due to deaths being allocated to alternative diagnoses. The great variations in incidence between and within countries and the remarkable changes in mortality in some countries within a relatively short period of time suggest that environmental factors play a major role.

Risk factors

While the ultimate causes of coronary heart disease remain uncertain, epidemiological studies have implicated a number of risk factors. In most cases, multiple risk factors are probably involved, and it is only in exceptional cases that one can attribute the disease to a single specific factor.

Lipids Paramount amongst the factors is the plasma level of cholesterol, as coronary disease is relatively uncommon in populations in which the cholesterol level is low, even if the other risk factors such as cigarette smoking and hypertension, are present. The most important component of the plasma lipids in this regard is low density lipoprotein (LDL).[3] By contrast, high density lipoproteins (HDL) appear to have a protective effect. The importance of triglycerides is disputed, but it seems probable that they are a relatively minor risk factor except when combined with high LDL or a low HDL.

Smoking   Epidemiological surveys in many countries, but particularly in the UK, have confirmed the strong relationship between the number of cigarettes smoked and the incidence of coronary heart disease.[4] This relationship holds in countries with very different rates of coronary disease, but the impact of smoking appears to be much greater when the plasma cholesterol is raised. The risk of coronary disease gradually decreases over a period of years in those who have given up smoking (see Chapter 2).

Alcohol   Heavy drinkers have a higher risk of cardiovascular disease, but those who have a moderate intake suffer less coronary disease than non-drinkers. There is some evidence that light regular alcohol consumption is actually protective, but the issue remains controversial.

Hypertension   There is a strong relationship between the levels of both systolic and diastolic pressure and the incidence of coronary disease, but again this is influenced by the level of cholesterol in the community. Thus, in spite of a high prevalence of hypertension in the Japanese and Afro-caribbeans, coronary heart disease is relatively uncommon.

Coagulation factors   It has been shown that raised levels of certain coagulation factors have a high predictive value for coronary heart disease.[5] The factors most clearly identified are fibrinogen and active Factor VII.

Physical exercise   Although less well established (but more difficult to study) as a risk factor than hyperlipidaemia, hypertension and cigarette smoking, there is an impressive body of evidence suggesting that regular physical exercise protects against coronary disease.[6,7]

Obesity   There is a positive association between overweight and coronary heart disease, but it is not clear to what extent this is an independent factor, or operates through other mechanisms such as hypertension.

Other risk factors

A number of other risk factors have been identified in coronary heart disease, such as the use of oral contraceptives, and the presence of diabetes. Others, less well established, include personality type (Type A), dietary deficiences (eg fish, linoleic acid, vitamins C and E), soft water, etc. Almost certainly there are additional risk factors that have yet to be discovered. Thus, the high incidence of coronary heart disease in members of the South Asian community in this country is not adequately accounted for by the known factors, although some evidence points to insulin resistance.

Family history

Young victims of coronary heart disease often have a family history of heart disease or sudden death at a relatively young age. Some of these have an identifiable genetic defect, of which the best known is that of familial hypercholesterolaemia, which is due to a defect in the LDL receptor. This affects some 1 in 500 of the population, but it is likely that at least 1% of the population have some form of specific genetic defect leading to premature coronary disease. Most individuals who develop coronary heart disease have a combination of a number of genetic and environmental risk factors, none of which is extremely abnormal. The risk factors are multiplicative rather than purely additive; this is of particular relevance in those with familial disorders. It is sometimes assumed that little can be done to help them; on the contrary, the correction of the environmental factors is of especial importance to such individuals.

Methods and effects of treating risk factors

The best established risk factors of hyperlipidaemia, smoking and hypertension are all amenable to correction, as are some other factors such as overweight, lack of exercise, and the use of oral contraceptives. It is therefore reasonable to presume that coronary heart disease is, at least partly, preventable by changes in living habits supplemented, if necessary, by medical treatment. Unfortunately, the evidence to date is not completely convincing that control of any one of the risk factors is effective in reducing mortality.

Hyperlipidaemia Several trials of lipid-lowering agents (such as clofibrate, gemfibrozil, nicotinic acid, and cholestyramine) have shown a reduction in coronary events, including cardiac death and non-fatal myocardial infarction.[8] In none of these studies has there been a significant reduction in total mortality; indeed in a WHO trial with clofibrate, there was a significant increase in total mortality in the treated group. The failure to demonstrate a reduction in total mortality could be a function of inadequate sample size in the studies, but might be due to adverse non-cardiac effects of the drugs counteracting a cardiac benefit. The extent of lipid-lowering in all the studies to date has, however, been modest; it will be of great interest to observe the effect on all cause mortality of the HMG CoA reductase inhibitors* since their effectiveness as lipid-lowering agents greatly exceeds that of the other drugs in current use.

Few studies have examined the effect of diet on coronary events and the difficulties of conducting such experiments are great. It is doubtful if trials which demonstrate the effects of changes in diet will ever be possible because of the difficulty of controlling for items of diet, because of the very large numbers of individuals who would have to be studied, and because of the need for decades of follow-up.

In spite of the inadequacy of the data, there is a strong argument for encouraging changes in the diet that will lead to a reduction in LDL cholesterol (see also Chapter 4). Some concern has been expressed as to whether it is wise to lower cholesterol substantially in those who have become habituated to a high level, and it has been suggested that lowering cholesterol might lead to cancer. The evidence for this is far from convincing, although the possibility cannot be totally dismissed at present. There is no reason to suppose, however, that there are dangers for young people who have not as yet become hypercholestero-laemic in taking a diet aimed at maintaining a low cholesterol level; thus, there is little or no evidence of an excess of cancers in those countries in which cholesterol levels in the community are low. It, therefore, appears prudent, particularly in the young, to discourage those foods, especially saturated fats, that lead to hyperlipidaemia. It also seems wise to encourage the consumption of fish, fruit and green vegetables. The consumption of fibre may lead to a reduction in plasma cholesterol, and such foods as oats and beans may be valuable in this context (see Chapter 3).

The role of drugs in the management of hyperlipidaemia remains to be clarified. As mentioned above, it appears that lipid-lowering drugs can reduce the incidence of coronary events, but their long-term safety record is still not established, particularly with the newer and more effective compounds. Short-term safety, however, appears to be good and it is reasonable to administer such agents to those with very high lipid levels or less high levels if other risk factors are present. The

---

*3-Hydroxy 3-methylglutaryl co-enzyme A (HMG CoA) reductase catalyses an important step in cholesterol synthesis. Competitive inhibitors of this enzyme, by reducing intracellular cholesterol, induce an increase of receptors for low density lipoprotein (LDL) in the liver, which results in lowering of total and LDL cholesterol in the plasma.

definition of 'high' is open to debate. The British Cardiac Society[9] suggested that drugs should be considered if the plasma cholesterol was above 7.8 mmol/l, whereas the European Atherosclerosis Society[10] proposed the optional use of lipid-lowering agents if the cholesterol was above 6.5 mmol/l. In both reports, it was emphasised that other risk factors and other features of the lipid profile should be taken into account in deciding upon drug treatment.

Smoking Satisfactory controlled trials of smoking cessation are almost impossible to organise, but there is much circumstantial evidence that stopping smoking diminishes the risk of heart disease. It may take some years to have an appreciable effect in the apparently normal population but seems to have a more immediate benefit in those who have already sustained a heart attack.

Hypertension Although the relationship between blood pressure and the incidence of coronary heart disease seems clear-cut, trials of anti-hypertensive treatment have been disappointing in showing little reduction in its incidence. It may be that the duration of the trials was too short, or that the number of events was too small to show a benefit. It is also possible that a potential benefit was being counteracted by adverse effects. For example, several antihypertensive agents increase lipid levels, or there may be an adverse effect on blood flow to the heart muscle if blood pressure is lowered too much.

Coagulation factors The only evidence that the treatment of haematological factors affects the incidence of coronary heart disease relates to the use of aspirin. The US Physicians primary prevention study[11] suggests that the regular consumption in a dosage of 160 mg a day reduces the risk of myocardial infarction. The case for aspirin is unequivocal in secondary prevention; it is clear that aspirin lessens the chance of re-infarction in those who have already sustained myocardial infarction or have unstable angina. Because aspirin may cause bleeding of the gastrointestinal tract or other organs, this risk albeit small makes it unwise to recommend its use in primary prevention in low risk groups.

Hormone replacement therapy There is some evidence that oestrogen therapy reduces the incidence of coronary disease in the post-menopausal woman. Whether combined oestrogen/progestogen therapy has the same beneficial effect is unknown.

Why is the incidence of coronary heart disease changing in some countries?

There has been a very remarkable reduction in deaths attributed to coronary heart disease in some countries, but not in others[12] (Fig. 5.2). The most striking changes have taken place in the United States and

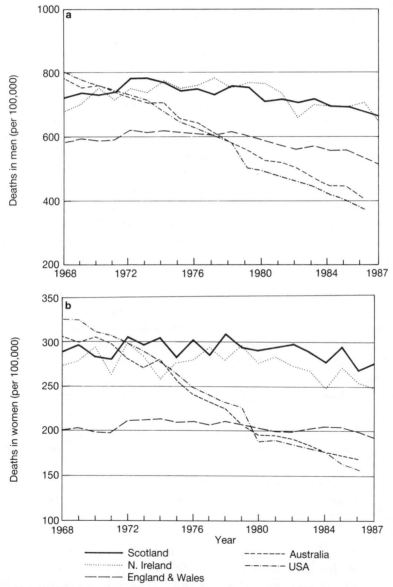

Fig. 5.2 *Death rates from coronary heart disease by country 1968–87: (a) men aged 35–74; (b) women aged 35–74.* Source: *Coronary Prevention Group/British Heart Foundation (1988)* Statistical information on coronary heart disease.

Table 5.1 Mortality reduction from peak for men aged 35–74 years, 1968–1987.

Age	England & Wales	USA
35–44	44%	63%
45–54	37%	53%
55–64	20%	56%
65–74	17%	54%

Australia, but reductions have also been encountered in Canada, New Zealand, Belgium, the Netherlands, Finland and Japan. In the USA, age standardised (35–74) death rates for males were 800 in 1968 and 375 in 1986. The comparable figures for Australia were 779 and 405, and in England and Wales 583 and 439.

A notable feature of the trends in England and Wales has been the much greater reduction in mortality among men in the younger age groups compared with the older; the difference between the age groups is much less marked in the United States (Table 5.1).

It is noteworthy that in spite of the impressive changes in the United States and Australia, the age-standardised mortality rates per 100,000 men in these countries remain high compared with Japan (64 in 1986), France (163) and Belgium (257). Epidemiologists have sought to explain these differences, and most have related them to diet, particularly the relatively low consumption of saturated fat, high polyunsaturated/saturated ratio and low cholesterol levels in Japan. There is some evidence that cholesterol levels have become lower in the USA and Australia in recent years. The consumption of saturated fat has not, however, fallen in the USA, but that of polyunsaturates has considerably increased.

It is probable that the large reductions in mortality that have occurred in some countries are indeed due to lifestyle changes. These countries have had the most vigorous programmes of 'coronary prevention' but they have also had the best provision of cardiac treatment services including surgery. The falls in mortality are, however, of a much greater magnitude than could be fully explained by treatment interventions.

It is likely that what improvement has taken place in the UK in recent years has been associated with the reduction in cigarette smoking, because the greatest fall in deaths from ischaemic heart disease has taken place in the social groups in whom reduction in cigarette smoking has been greatest.

Policies for preventive action

Two approaches to prevention have been proposed which have been termed the *high-risk* strategy and the *population* strategy:

- The *high risk strategy* requires the identification and treatment of individuals at high risk of coronary heart disease. This demands considerable effort and expense involving screening by clinical examination and laboratory investigations. For the individuals identified, however, it is probably of great value, allowing the targeting of specific therapy.

- The *population strategy* is based on the knowledge that in countries such as the UK a high percentage of the population exhibit one or more of the risk factors. For this reason, a major impact on the incidence of coronary heart disease can be made only if preventive measures are applied to most of the population; it seems likely that changes in diet, smoking habit, and exercise, and the treatment of hypertension would yield a considerable reduction in mortality from coronary disease.

The high risk and population strategies have sometimes been cast as opposites but they can be complementary; there is no reason why both should not be implemented.

Screening for raised levels of plasma cholesterol

Plasma cholesterol can now be measured relatively simply and cheaply, and in some countries, notably the United States, it is recommended that all members of the public should 'know their number'. Demand for cholesterol screening has become widespread in the UK, and cholesterol tests are available from a number of different sources, including pharmacists, private health organisations, and food health stores, as well as some general practitioners. Those who have their cholesterol measured need to be made aware of the other risk factors for coronary heart disease, because the significance of a particular cholesterol level depends upon these, being of little importance if no other risk factors are present. Skilled professional counselling must be readily available to those having their cholesterol measured, both to explain the implications of the findings, and to advise on diet or further investigation, as necessary.

Mass screening for cholesterol is a controversial and complex issue. The main *arguments in favour* of it are that:

1. Only in this way may those with very high lipids (eg those with familial hyperlipidaemia) be identified.

2. A knowledge of one's cholesterol level is a motivator leading to a beneficial change in diet.

Arguments against mass screening are that:

1. While it is important to identify those with familial disorders, many of the affected individuals can be identified simply by taking a family history because premature coronary disease has occurred in members of their families.
2. It has not been clearly established that a knowledge of one's cholesterol level does act as an effective motivator. This information may, on the other hand, cause unnecessary anxiety.
3. Cholesterol levels are variable within an individual and abnormal cholesterol measurements need to be repeated, and may require further investigation by a detailed lipid analysis to determine LDL and HDL levels.
4. The measurement of cholesterol is subject to inaccuracies. This is particularly true where blood sampling and laboratory testing are not under stringent supervision.
5. Positive results of cholesterol measurement must be followed by counselling. The expense of a mass cholesterol screening programme is, therefore, much greater than that of simply carrying out cheap tests on everyone.
6. Raised plasma cholesterol is only one of the risk factors for coronary heart disease, and carries little prognostic weight if no other factors are present. A relatively low plasma cholesterol may imply, wrongly, that the individual is not at risk of coronary disease. Thus, cholesterol level on its own is a screening test with both poor sensitivity and poor specificity for subsequent myocardial infarction.

In May 1990, the Standing Medical Advisory Committee reported to the Secretary of State for Health on *Blood cholesterol testing — the cost-effectiveness of opportunistic cholesterol screening*. The essential conclusion (7.3.3 of the Report) was that:

> the most cost-effective approach involves an opportunistic programme in which coronary heart disease risk factors are identified, priority being given to plasma cholesterol measurement in individuals of high overall risk of coronary heart disease. The groups at highest risk of coronary heart disease mortality include persons with existing coronary heart disease, those with risk factors such as elevated blood pressure, cigarette smoking and diabetes, and those with a family history of coronary heart disease or hyperlipidaemia. Individuals with more than one risk factor for coronary heart disease should be given priority over those with one known risk factor, and the latter should receive priority over those with no known risk factor.

These conclusions are in broad agreement with those of the King's Fund Consensus Statement on *Blood Cholesterol Measurement in the prevention of Coronary Heart Disease* and the policy of a number of medical organisations concerned with the prevention of coronary heart disease. There is, therefore, a widely held view in the UK that there should be opportunistic plasma cholesterol measurements of *selected* groups in the population, as opposed to the essentially unselected screening of adults for hypertension.

Hypertension

Hypertension is a major risk factor for both coronary heart disease and stroke,[13] but its relationship to stroke is of particular importance because it is the major identifiable risk factor, and because anti-hypertensive treatment has been demonstrated to be highly effective in stroke prevention.[14]

Prevention of hypertension

The environmental factors involved in the development of hypertension are not well-defined, but increased weight and excessive alcohol are common contributors. The role of salt is not so firmly established, although the weight of evidence suggests that high intakes can cause hypertension in susceptible individuals and that low intakes protect against it. Other possible factors include sedentary lifestyle, inadequate potassium and magnesium intake, exposure to lead and cadmium, disturbances of calcium metabolism, and stress and noise.

In practical terms the best established methods of prevention seem to be:

- avoidance of overweight,
- avoidance of excessive consumption of alcohol,
- restriction of salt, and
- regular physical exercise.

Screening for hypertension

Hypertension is frequently not recognised until one of its major complications, such as stroke or myocardial infarction, has occurred. It seldom gives rise to symptoms and its satisfactory control depends upon its identification in the asymptomatic population.

It is generally accepted that hypertension should be detected by the opportunistic recording of the blood pressure by the primary health care team; this should be undertaken at intervals of not more than 5 years in all adults. Unfortunately, this is not sufficiently widely practised, and many cases go undetected until complications occur. Occupational health services and other medical facilities (including surgical wards and antenatal clinics) can make an important contribution to the detection of hypertension.

Treatment

Clinical trials have established that antihypertensive treatment is effective in the prevention of stroke,[14] but the precise indications for such treatment remain uncertain. While it can be shown, as in the MRC trial,[15] that lowering blood pressure has an effect in the prevention of stroke in mild hypertension, the absolute benefit is small and the cost-benefit ratio a matter of discussion. Guidelines on the indications for treatment of mild hypertension have recently been published in a memorandum from a World Health Organisation/International Society of Hypertension meeting.[16]

Relaxation programmes, yoga, transcendental meditation and biofeedback all seem to reverse mild hypertension in the short term, but their long-term effectiveness has yet to be established.

The drug treatment of hypertension is beyond the scope of this report, but it should be mentioned that, because of the differing metabolic effect of the various categories of drug, the choice of agent may be important.

Stroke

Causes of stroke

Some 80% of strokes result from cerebral infarction and 10% each from subarachnoid haemorrhage and primary intracerebral haemorrhage. As already seen, the major risk factor for cerebral infarction and primary cerebral haemorrhage is hypertension. Other identified risk factors include obesity, oral contraceptives, excessive alcohol consumption, diabetes mellitus and a high haematocrit. Although cigarette smoking is not an important risk factor for hypertension, it increases the risk of complications, including stroke. Cerebral embolism resulting from cardiac disorders, such as atrial fibrillation, myocardial infarction and mitral valve prolapse is responsible for perhaps 10–15% of all strokes.

Prevention of stroke

The prevention of stroke largely depends upon the control of hypertension. Aspirin and anticoagulants are valuable in the prevention of cerebral emboli resulting from pre-existing cardiac disease. Although aspirin has been shown to prevent the development of stroke in those who have already suffered from transient ischaemic attacks, it seems probable that it can occasionally cause cerebral haemorrhage. It should be used with caution in those with hypertension, and should not be used routinely for the prevention of stroke in apparently healthy normal individuals.

The prevention of other cardiac disorders

Congenital heart disease   Congenital heart disease affects about eight in every 1,000 children born. In spite of the successes of surgery it still exerts a substantial toll of mortality and morbidity. Its causes are largely unknown, but rubella vaccination, and the avoidance of certain drugs may reduce the numbers of children born with serious disorders. In future, the use of fetal echocardiography to detect irreparable defects may enable termination of affected pregnancies.

Rheumatic heart disease   Rheumatic fever and its sequelae of valvular heart disease are now rare amongst those born in the United Kingdom, but they are not infrequent in the immigrant population. The decline in prevalence is probably due to a reduction in streptococcal infections largely brought about by improvements in social conditions, notably housing. Streptococcal infection, leading to recurrences of rheumatic fever and often to more heart damage, can be prevented by the use of long-term penicillin administration in patients with known rheumatic heart disease.

Infective endocarditis   This disorder still exacts a mortality in spite of the effectiveness of prompt antibiotic treatment. Unfortunately, many cardiac lesions are unrecognised until the patient presents with the manifestations of endocarditis. Nonetheless, some patients known to have congenital and valvular heart disease develop the infection because of ignorance on the part of the patient or inaction on the part of the doctor or dentist. All patients at risk should be impressed with the importance of dental hygiene and of informing their GP and dentist of their condition, and should carry a card which describes the cardiac problem and provides guidance on prevention of endocarditis. When possible, the cardiac defect (eg a persistent ductus arteriosus) should be corrected, but this is not always feasible and indeed, surgical treatment, as with the insertion of a prosthetic valve, may increase the risk of endocarditis.

Cardiomyopathies   The causes of cardiomyopathy are largely unknown, but it may be possible to prevent those which are due to alcohol and certain drugs (such as adriamycin).

RECOMMENDATIONS

The Recommendations of Chapters 2, 3 and 4 are all relevant to reduction of cardiovascular disease. In addition:

1   The detection and treatment of hypertension is important in the prevention of stroke, and of cardiac and renal failure, and, to a lesser extent, in the prevention of coronary heart disease. The blood pressure should be checked by the primary health care team at least every five years in every adult. This is a requirement of the new general practitioner contract.

2   Physical exercise should be encouraged, and facilities for the cheap but excellent forms of exercise such as cycling and swimming should be improved to the levels available in comparable countries abroad. Places of work should, if possible, provide time and facilities for this purpose.

3   General practitioners and the primary care health team play a key role in the prevention of coronary heart disease. It is desirable that all patients should be periodically checked for risk factors for coronary heart disease, and appropriate further measures taken (eg counselling, reference to hospital, or cholesterol measurement), as necessary.

4   Attempts should be made to identify individuals with an inherited susceptibility to coronary heart disease. This requires action on the part of hospital physicians and general practitioners to investigate the close relatives of patients who present with coronary heart disease at an early age.

5   Mass cholesterol screening is not recommended as a means of prevention at the present time, but plasma cholesterol should be measured in those with a family history of premature coronary heart disease (defined as below age 50 in men and 55 in women), those with moderate or severe hypertension, and those who smoke, or have other risk factors such as diabetes. Further lipid studies may be undertaken, if indicated in those with raised plasma cholesterol.

7   Doctors in general, and cardiologists in particular, should become better informed about and take a more active interest in preventive aspects.

8   Much further research needs to be undertaken into the causes and prevention of coronary heart disease and hypertension, and into the best ways of implementing the knowledge already available.

6 Cancer

Cancer is responsible for around 25% of deaths in the UK; around one-third of individuals will develop some form of cancer during their lifetime. It is now generally accepted that whilst cancer is not completely preventable the great majority of cancers could in theory be avoided. The incidence of most cancers varies greatly between parts of the world with different lifestyles and environments. For each cancer, if the lowest incidence reported from any country with reliable data pertained in all countries, then the total world burden of cancer would be reduced by 80–90%. Many causes of cancer have now been identified, including environmental carcinogens, intrinsic factors such as hormonal imbalances, viral infections, reproductive activities, and a variety of other factors which depend to some extent on personal behaviour.

Evidence for preventability of cancer

Evidence that much human cancer is potentially avoidable is contained within four main categories and can be summarised as:

- differences in the incidence of cancer between different countries and communities;
- differences between migrants from a particular community and those who remain behind;
- variations over time in the incidence of cancer;
- identification of specific causal or preventive factors.[1]

International comparisons show that in the case of several cancers the range between countries with the highest and lowest incidence may be a hundred-fold or more. Many other common cancer rates vary by lesser, but still very appreciable amounts. Studies of Japanese who have migrated to Hawaii have shown that their cancer rates are more like those for Caucasian residents of Hawaii than for Japanese in Japan. Thus, the rates of colon and rectal cancer are much higher in Japanese in Hawaii than in those in Japan. There is also a four-fold increase in breast cancer incidence. By contrast, stomach cancer is much less common in Japanese in Hawaii than in those in Japan.

Within the UK in this century there has been a large increase in cancer caused almost entirely by the increase in lung cancer. However, the overall cancer death rate is levelling off, and when age-specific rates are examined over time one can see that the risk of dying from cancer is decreasing in successive generations. Overall, cancer mortality in those aged between 20 and 45 has fallen by 40% in males and 30% in females since the 1950s, but it remains to be seen whether this decreased risk will be sustained as the present generation gets older. Although some part of the improvement in death rate is due to more successful treatment for those cancers that affect young people, the greater part is due to decreasing incidence, as evidenced by trends in incidence shown by the national cancer registration scheme. The decreasing overall incidence is dominated by a recent fall in lung cancer (see Chapter 2) and a longer term decrease in stomach cancer. Apart from these two major sites, overall incidence is increasing, particularly in the elderly.[2] Moreover, because cancer is more common in the elderly and the proportion of elderly in the population is going to increase for the next 20 years, a further increase in the number of cancer deaths can be anticipated.

As already mentioned, there are marked changes in incidence for cancers of different sites. By far the greatest part of the increase this century has been from lung cancer which in men started to rise in the 1920s, reached a peak in the 1960s, then plateaued and has now begun to fall. A similar trend has occurred in women but starting 20 years later and only very recently starting to plateau. Age-specific rates for men at all ages under 85 years are falling. For men under the age of 50 they have now fallen substantially and are beginning to do so also in young women. In spite of these recent declines, lung cancer still accounts for more deaths than any other cancer site in men, and among women is rapidly overtaking breast cancer as the leading cause of cancer death.

Other sites in which incidence and mortality are increasing include malignant melanoma of the skin, non-Hodgkin's lymphoma, multiple myeloma and breast cancer. Cervical cancer mortality has fallen very slightly, but within this overall picture there has been a substantial reduction among women aged 40 and over, offset by an increase in younger women in recent years. Testicular cancer is rising in incidence, but due to the success of treatment there is an increasing gap between incidence and mortality, which is now falling. In common with many other countries, stomach cancer, although still common, is falling in incidence and mortality.

There is overwhelming evidence for a number of factors in the causation of cancer (Table 6.1) and some evidence that other factors are also involved (Table 6.2). Exposure to most of these causes of cancer can be controlled to some extent by individuals. It is therefore

Table 6.1 Proven causes of cancer of importance in UK (excluding occupational hazards)

Cause	Type of cancer
Tobacco smoking*	Lung, larynx, lip, mouth, pharynx, oesophagus, pancreas, bladder, renal pelvis
Over-nutrition leading to obesity	Gall-bladder, endometrium
Alcoholic drinks[+]	Mouth, pharynx, oesophagus, larynx, liver
Tobacco chewing	Mouth
Ionising radiation (radon in houses)	Lung
Ultraviolet light	Melanoma, squamous and basal cell skin cancers
Hepatitis B virus	Liver
Sexual activity (? some types of human papilloma virus)	Cervix, anus, penis
Low parity	Ovary
Late age at first birth	Breast
Unopposed oestrogens	Endometrium, breast

*Possibly also contributing to cancers of body of kidney, cervix, stomach, liver, leukaemia and nasal sinuses.
[+]Possibly also contributing to cancers of breast and (beer only) rectum.

Table 6.2   Suspected causes of cancer of importance in UK

Deficiency of:

Fruit	Stomach
Green vegetables	Stomach, large bowel
Beta-carotene	Most carcinomas
Fibre and resistant starch	Large bowel

Excess of:

Fat (possibly excluding olive oil)	Breast, large bowel, prostate
Salt preserved foods	Stomach

important that all doctors should be able to advise and educate their patients and the public on what steps can be taken to avoid cancer, how much this will reduce their risk of cancer, and what good or bad side-effects the action might have.

Risk factors

Tobacco

Around 40,000 UK residents and 400,000 Europeans die from cancer due to smoking every year.[3] Smoking is responsible for around one third of all cancer deaths in some countries. The commonest site is, of course, the lung, and others include the lip, oral cavity, pharynx, larynx, oesophagus, bladder, kidney, pancreas, and possibly, cervix and bone marrow. That smoking can cause so many cancers at different sites is understandable because of the presence in tobacco smoke of many different carcinogens. Tobacco smoke is more harmful in the form of cigarettes than when smoked in pipes or cigars, and tends to cause cancer after regular exposure for 30 to 40 years. **The risk of lung cancer among people who smoke 20 or more cigarettes a day for many years is 20 times that of non-smokers, and cigarette-smoking accounts for over 90% of all lung cancers**. There is good evidence that reducing tar levels in cigarettes results in a reduction in mortality from lung cancer, but low tar cigarettes may not have any effect on the incidence of cancers that result from the absorption of carcinogens into the blood stream, or on other smoking-related conditions such as coronary heart disease. Passive smoking—inhalation by non-smokers of other people's cigarette smoke—is also associated with a slightly increased risk of lung cancer but the risk for non-smokers is low and the increase slight (relative risk up to 1.5), so that this is not a major cause of lung cancer. Tobacco chewing rather than smoking, as in products such as Skoal Bandits, is also dangerous because it may lead to cancer of the mouth. In 1990, manufacture and sale of these products were banned in the UK but, because of legal technicalities, an appeal by the manufacturers was upheld by a High Court. Although the ban remains at least temporarily in force the final outcome is uncertain. Guidance on the most effective methods for helping patients stop smoking is given in Chapter 2.

Dietary factors and cancer

There is substantial evidence that diet can influence the incidence of cancer and it is likely that the risk of cancer could be substantially reduced by dietary modification.[4] Furthermore, many of the suggested changes are entirely consistent with recommendations aimed at preventing other major diseases, such as ischaemic heart disease (see Chapters 4 and 5).

There is good evidence that *reduction of obesity* should lead to a reduction of cancer of the gall-bladder and of the body of uterus.[5] A number of case-control and cohort studies have suggested a protective effect from the consumption of *fruit* and *green vegetables* on stomach cancer and green vegetables and *fibre* on cancers of the lower gastro-intestinal tract. The mechanisms by which these factors exert their effects is not clear. Assessment of the role of dietary fibre, for instance, is complicated by uncertainty about the components of fibre which might exert beneficial effects, and the benefit may merely be related to the ability of fibre to reach the large bowel and provide a substrate for bacteria. In the case of fruit, vitamin C could be an active component against nitrite in the stomach but whether nitrate is important is not certain. Amongst green vegetables, cabbage, brussels sprouts and other members of the cruciferae family may be particularly effective. The methodological problems in determining the mechanisms by which diet may prevent cancer, and the duration of time between dietary deficiency (or excess) and development of cancer, have inhibited experimental trials in which people without cancer are allocated to eat or not to eat certain foods. Because experimental evidence is lacking, the reduction in risk which would follow adherence to a diet with specified amounts of these ingredients is not known, but advice to eat them at least several times a week is reasonable.

A considerable number of studies have now shown that blood levels of *beta-carotene, selenium* and *vitamin E* have been, on average, lower in patients who went on to develop cancer than in controls. The strongest evidence probably relates to beta-carotene. For none of these constituents, however, is the current evidence strong enough for increasing consumption to be unequivocally advocated. Beta-carotene is currently being tested in a randomised controlled trial among US doctors.

Many epidemiological and laboratory studies have been conducted to examine the association between cancer and *dietary lipids*. There are strong international correlations between dietary fat intake and cancer at several sites, including breast, large bowel and prostate, although it is difficult to separate national fat consumption from other aspects of a high standard of living. At an individual level it is difficult to obtain precise estimates of fat consumption, and case-control and cohort studies have given conflicting results. There is a theory that polyunsaturates might be more likely to produce cancer, possibly because of an association with free radical formation, but the evidence is inconclusive. Overall, there is unsufficient evidence to recommend reducing fat consumption purely with the aim of reducing the risk of cancer.

A range of other dietary measures have been suggested by various investigators to have an impact on cancer, but the evidence for most of these factors, which include avoidance of nitrates, saccharine, salt-preserved food, smoked and grilled fish, is not conclusive enough to permit firm recommendations. An increase in the consumption of fruit and green vegetables can, however, be confidently advised.

Alcohol

There is firm evidence from a range of studies that alcohol is related to cancer at several sites. In many cases, the effect appears to be synergistic with cigarette smoking; in one study, cancer of the oesophagus was found to be 90 times more common in those who drank alcohol heavily and smoked heavily, than in non-drinkers and non-smokers. Alcohol is a contributory cause of cancers of mouth, pharynx, larynx, oesophagus and liver. Alcohol is also associated with breast cancer and large bowel cancer. These associations support the need to restrict alcohol consumption as recommended in Chapter 3.

Ionising radiation

There is still some uncertainty about the magnitude of the long-term carcinogenic effect of ionising radiation at very low levels. Recently, revised estimates of dose received by the survivors of Hiroshima and Nagasaki atomic bombs, and more prolonged observation of the survivors, have suggested an effect for high levels of exposure some two to five times greater than previously thought.

The two main sources of radiation which may be, at least in part, preventable, are natural radon gas in domestic buildings, and medical X-ray examinations.

Radon   is a radioactive gas naturally emitted from granite rock, and is therefore found mainly in geologically defined parts of the country, such as Cornwall and Devon. In the past, it had been thought to make only a small contribution to risk of cancer but it has now been realised that the concentration of the gas can build up to levels at which prolonged inhalation can lead to lung cancer. Moreover, it is thought that it acts synergistically with cigarette smoking. If the concentration of radon in a house is above 200 becquerels per cubic metre of air, it is estimated that the life-time risk of dying from lung cancer is 1% for non-smokers and 10% for smokers; this implies approximately 2,500 lung cancer deaths each year. Action to reduce radon concentration by installing underfloor ventilation is recommended for houses with concentrations above 200 becquerels per cubic metre. These are likely to occur in Cornwall and Devon (12% of homes), Somerset, Northamptonshire and Derby (1% of homes) and Grampian, Highland and South West Scotland (1% of homes). The National Radiological Protection Board provides advice on radon measurement.

Medical diagnostic and therapeutic X-rays   employ modern techniques aimed at minimising dose and targeting the relevant part of the body. The risk of cancer induced by medical X-rays is therefore minuscule compared to their value in management of disease. Nevertheless, radiation doses from medical equipment are regularly monitored. It is important that clinicians should avoid ordering even simple investigations such as chest X-rays unless the X-ray is medically justified; particular care needs to be taken in ordering X-rays for pregnant women and young children. Unfortunately, there has recently been an increasing tendency for X-rays to be taken in order to protect the doctor from medical litigation, even when such investigations are not necessarily in the best interests of the patients concerned: more attention needs to be paid to developing agreed policies which will diminish this trend towards unnecessary and possibly harmful investigation.

Nuclear installations

Workers in the nuclear industries are subject to stringent controls on their exposure. Concern about leukaemia, and other cancer risks, among people living close to nuclear plants is widespread. The question of increased risk around some nuclear installations is, however, still unresolved and is the subject of ongoing research. It is noteworthy that the public fear of radiation is out of all proportion to public fear about much more hazardous carcinogens such as tobacco.

Ultraviolet radiation

There has been increasing interest in the relationship between sunlight and skin cancer, particularly in view of the threat of ozone depletion in the atmosphere resulting from increasing use of chlorofluorocarbons (CFCs) and other pollutants. Basal cell and squamous cell carcinomas are associated with long-term cumulative exposure to natural sunlight, and are commoner in those with occupational exposure, such as farmers and fishermen. These tumours have an excellent prognosis so that, although their incidence is high, mortality is almost negligible. Malignant melanoma of the skin is less common but accounts for the great majority of deaths from skin cancer. A number of studies have shown that fair-skinned individuals who tend to burn easily, have difficulty in tanning, have light coloured hair, skin and eyes, and who have increased numbers of benign pigmented naevi (moles), have a greater risk of melanoma than dark-skinned people. Both incidence and mortality have been increasing in many countries, and it is thought that this results from a change in sun-bathing habits over the past two decades. Office workers who spend most of their working life indoors but who are exposed to sunlight episodically on holiday are at greater risk than those who are regularly exposed. A history of severe sunburn, particularly in childhood, also appears to increase the risk of melanoma. Patients with previously diagnosed dysplastic naevus syndrome (ie who have considerable numbers of pigmented naevi which are usually large and may have an irregular edge and look inflamed) are also at high risk.

There is circumstantial evidence to suggest that advice to avoid excessive exposure to sun reduces melanoma incidence. In Queensland, Australia, which has the highest rates in the world and which has had a vigorous public campaign for several years (SLIP on a T-shirt, SLAP on a hat, and SLOP on protective sun-cream), the incidence of melanoma in children seems to have begun to decline. Nevertheless, experimental evidence is still lacking. Similarly, although advice to people on early detection of malignant melanoma, and immediate reporting of suspicious signs, is reasonable, there is no evidence as yet that public education about early detection has any effect on the death rate.

It is important for all doctors, especially those in general practice, to be aware of the seven signs of malignant melanoma (itch, diameter greater than 1 cm, increasing size, irregular border, vaiable pigment density, inflammation and crusting) and of the need to refer patients with four or more of these characteristics to a dermatologist.[6]

Occupational carcinogens

Cancers caused by known occupational carcinogens probably represent a relatively small proportion of all cancer cases. In the US, it has been calculated as around 4% of all cancer deaths. The main cancers concerned are lung cancer among workers exposed to asbestos and various metallic products such as *chromates*; bladder cancer among those exposed to aromatic amines in the *rubber* and *dye* industries; angiosarcoma of the liver in those exposed to *vinyl chloride*; and various cancers in those exposed to ionizing radiation (see Chapter 10).

The most comprehensive list of known carcinogens to which individuals can be exposed at work comes from the International Agency for Research on Cancer (IARC).[7] A total of 628 agents have been evaluated for evidence of carcinogenicity before 1988, of which 246 were classified as carcinogenic or possibly carcinogenic to humans. Of the agents, 101 are industrial chemicals, 13 are pesticides, 49 laboratory chemicals and 58 drugs are also implicated. An EC directive on labelling chemical compounds for carcinogenicity was issued in 1983. Substances which are known to be carcinogenic, or those which should be regarded as if they are carcinogenic to man, should be labelled with the phrase 'R45 *may cause cancer*'. Substances with possible carcinogenic effects are to be labelled 'R40 *possible risk of irreversible effects*'. Mutagenicity testing has been required for all new chemicals marketed in the EC since 1980. The number that has actually been shown to cause cancer in humans is small and a large proportion of these are drugs that are used for the treatment of cancer.

Non-occupational asbestos

Asbestos has become very widespread in our environment and studies in occupational groups have indicated that those exposed to the fibres of some forms of asbestos have an increased risk of mesothelioma, a characteristic tumour of the pleura or peritoneum, and of carcinoma of the lung. Mesothelioma is particularly associated with crocidolite and amosite. The third form of asbestos, chrysolite seldom causes mesothelioma and may have to continue to be used under controlled conditions until the safety of potential substitutes has been demonstrated. The risk of cancer from non-occupational sources of exposure is very small and removal of asbestos already in place (for example in ceiling insulation) is likely to cause greater hazard than leaving it alone.[8] But public anxiety about the carcinogenic effect of asbestos has overridden scientific advice, and demand for asbestos removal continues.

Viruses and cancer

Several oncogenic viruses have been incriminated as causes of cancer. Worldwide the most important is the *hepatitis B virus (HBV)* which leads to primary liver carcinoma among chronically infected people with HBV; this is the commonest cancer in men in many parts of the developing world. Not all those infected go on to develop carcinoma and it may be that further exposure to another carcinogenic agent (possibly aflatoxin) is also required. Immunisation against HBV should offer protection against the cancer (as well as hepatitis) and long-term trials have been set up in West Africa and the Far East to test this hypothesis.

Another oncogenic virus of importance in these countries, but not the UK, is the *Epstein Barr virus*, causing nasopharyngeal tumours in China and Burkitt's lymphoma in Africa.

Human papilloma virus (HPV)   HPV appears to be closely related to cancers of the cervix and probably also penis and anus. However there are many different subtypes and only some of these appear to cause cancer. Moreover not all cervices infected with these subtypes develop cancer and it may be that, as with liver cancer, a further carcinogenic stimulus—possibly another virus such as herpes simplex type 2—is required. There is no vaccine yet available against HPV. This means that prevention of cervical, penile and anal cancers depends upon limiting the opportunities for infection. The current health education campaign to avoid HIV infection by use of condoms and restricting the number of sexual partners should have spin-off benefits in preventing these cancers.

Human immunodeficiency virus (HIV)   HIV infection is associated with Kaposi's sarcoma of the skin and gastrointestinal tract. Working through an immuno-suppressive effect the incidence of some other cancers is also raised in HIV-infected patients.

Exogenous oestrogens

The effects of *hormonal contraceptives* on breast cancer incidence have been intensively studied. No excess risk occurs among women who first use oral contraceptives in their late twenties or thirties after they have had children. However, most studies in younger women have found that those who have used oral contraceptives at young ages have a slight excess risk of breast cancer (relative risk about 1.5) at least up to age 45. Whether or not this higher risk will be sustained for the rest of life is not yet known. Oral contraceptives have also been implicated as a cause of cervical cancer but this may be only because both cervical cancer and use of oral contraceptives are indicators of sexual activity. Oral contraceptives have a protective effect against ovarian cancer and endometrial cancer, with 5 or more years' use of contraception halving risk up to age 55, this decreased risk being sustained for at least 10 years, and probably for the remainder of life.

By contrast, *postmenopausal hormone replacement therapy* with unopposed oestrogens increases risk of endometrial cancer, and possibly also breast cancer. When combined with progesterone, risk of endometrial cancer is reduced.

When advising women about use of these drugs, the possibilities of cancer induction and cancer reduction need to be explained and taken into account with other risks and other benefits specific to each individual woman's circumstances (eg need to avoid pregnancy, smoking habit, blood pressure). On present evidence it seems that, taking only cancers into account, the risks and benefits of oral contraception may cancel each other out; for HRT the cancer risks are greater than the cancer benefits but other benefits in prevention of osteoporosis and possibly ischaemic heart disease are considerable (see Chapter 11).

Screening for cancer

Screening aims to detect presymptomatic cancer at a stage in its natural history at which treatment will arrest its progression. For some cancers, tests are available which can detect possible malignancy even before it has become invasive, eg cervical intra-epithelial neoplasia, or premalignant adenomas of the large bowel. In these cases the success of screening can be judged by a reduction in the subsequent incidence of invasive cancer. For most cancers, however, screening is only able to detect the tumour when it is already invasive; here the hope is that early treatment will be curative. In these cases screening clearly cannot reduce incidence but is judged by a reduction in the subsequent death rate from the cancer.

Constraints to the success of screening

Screening cannot hope to be 100% successful in controlling any given cancer. There is always a range of progression rates, some cases spreading to the incurable stage so quickly that they could never be detected in time, while others may be so slow-growing that they are almost always curable. It is cases between these two extremes which can be favourably influenced by screening. Another constraint to the success of screening is that no test is 100% sensitive, meaning that some potentially detectable cancers will be missed. When the success of screening is judged on a population basis, as it has to be for unbiased comparison with a non-screening situation, further constraints are that not all the people offered screening will accept it (and those who do not accept are often those at greatest risk); and some cases of borderline malignancy may not be adequately followed up to definitive diagnosis and treatment.

Evaluating the effectiveness of screening

For many different cancer sites, screening tests have been shown to detect a *high yield of tumours* which have a more *favourable stage distribution* than those diagnosed through symptomatic presentation, and which also have *greatly improved survival rates*. While these three criteria—high prevalence, improved stage distribution and improved survival—are necessary concomitants of successful screening, they are insufficient evidence to prove that it is effective. In order to show experimentally whether or not screening reduces incidence or mortality it is necessary to compare a whole population for whom screening is available with a control population for whom it is not, over a period of several years from the introduction of the screening programme. Ideally, this comparison should take the form of a prospective randomised controlled trial, but where this is not possible because screening has already been provided on a service as opposed to research basis, retrospective evaluation can sometimes be done by relating trends in incidence or mortality to the intensity of screening, or by case-control studies to derive the relative protection afforded by screening.

Disadvantages of screening

Inevitably, the application of screening tests to large numbers of symptomless people has unwanted physical and psychological side-effects and a full evaluation should ideally weigh up the level of reduction in incidence and/or mortality against the disadvantages and costs. The disadvantages include:

- any possible hazard of the test itself,
- lack of specificity, and
- overdiagnosis.

The first is seldom a problem but nevertheless, because the test is to be applied to thousands of symptomless people, the vast majority of whom will derive no direct benefit, it is ethically very important to ensure that none of them are seriously harmed by it. *Lack of specificity* means that the test will give some false positive results requiring that these people have to undergo the anxiety and morbidity of further investigation, possibly requiring surgical biopsy, in order to eliminate the suspicion of cancer. *Specificity* is inversely related to sensitivity, so that a test designed to be highly sensitive will pick up virtually all early cancers but will also give many false positives, whereas a highly specific test gives very few false positive results, but may miss some cancers. Achieving a reasonable balance between sensitivity and specificity means that some false positives and some false negatives (missed cancers) have to be tolerated. Related to the problem of false positives is the potentially serious disadvantage of '*over-diagnosis*'. Screening inevitably picks up lesions of borderline histological neoplasia some of which will be malignant in their behaviour but others will be benign; because it is impossible to say which is which, all must be treated as possible cancers.

Costs

The *resource costs* of screening are also a considerable disadvantage, particularly since it needs to be regularly repeated over a long period to detect all newly arising cancers at a curable stage. When evaluating changes to a screening policy it is the *marginal costs* and benefits which are important, ie:

- How many extra deaths will be avoided by the policy change?
- How much extra will it cost?
- Is the cost of preventing these extra deaths the best use of these resources?

Sites of cancer screening

The scale and duration of research required to evaluate cancer screening accounts for the fact that, as yet, a clear answer on whether or not screening is worthwhile is only available for four cancer sites.

Cervical cancer

Screening, using cytological examination of a cervical smear, was introduced in the middle 1960s without any prior evaluation, and it has taken nearly 20 years to accumulate evidence of its effectiveness. Most of this has come from Scandinavia where different countries applied different screening policies, and where trends in incidence and mortality are published.[9] Finland, Iceland and Sweden, which had organised screening programmes reaching over 80% of women between 25 and 55–60, have achieved reductions in mortality of 50% or more, whereas in Denmark and Norway, where organised screening reached only 35% and 3% respectively of the target population, lesser changes (25% and 2% respectively) have occurred. Taking only women below age 35, however, there is little difference betwen the countries because much opportunistic screening is done in younger women, in association with consultations for contraception or antenatal care. This emphasises the point that opportunistic screening (as distinct from screening by invitation) may have some impact in young women but will fail to control cervical cancer adequately because the majority of cases, and the great majority of deaths, occur in women well beyond their child-bearing years.

Within the UK, over the same time period, trends in incidence and mortality have been similar to those of Norway. This apparent failure to have an effect has not been caused by lack of resources, since the number of smears examined each year is sufficient to screen all women 5-yearly, so much as by maldistribution of screening. Smears have been wastefully repeated with unnecessary frequency on young low-risk women and have failed to reach those most at risk. As with most cancers, risk increases with increasing age, and, because cervical cancer is almost certainly caused by a sexually transmitted viral infection, is more common in women with greater exposure to the risk of infection, namely those who themselves have had several sexual partners, or whose partners have had several partners. The lack of organisation of screening is highlighted by examining the screening history of women who develop invasive cancer. One study found that 66% had never been screened (90% in patients over 40), 15% had had inadequate follow-up of a mildly abnormal smear, 10% had not been screened for more than 5 years, and 9% had had a negative smear within 5 years of diagnosis.[10]

In recent years, as already seen, there has been an increase in incidence and mortality in women under the age of 35, probably associated with increasing risk of infection with HPV and/or other agents. It is almost certain that this increased risk will remain with this cohort of women as they grow older and, since incidence rises with increasing age, a large increase in cervical carcinoma can be anticipated, unless it is contained by organised screening of women of all age-groups. **It is therefore important to ensure that every woman over 20 is invited and encouraged to have a cervical smear at least once every 5 years**. Since 1988, a system of regular computerized invitations for every woman aged 20–65, registered with a general practitioner in England and Wales, has been started and it is hoped that this will correct the previous maldistribution of screening. It is however constrained by the inaccuracy of the patient registers held by Family Health Service Authorities, particularly in large conurbations. Most authorities suggest that screening is only necessary after age 65 for women who have not had two or more negative smears in the previous 10 years.

Costs: Extrapolating from case-control studies, it has been calculated that 5-yearly screening up to age 65 confers 84% protection against development of invasive cervical cancer; if the interval between routine repeat smears is shortened to 3-yearly, protection rises to 91%, and if shortened to annually protection rises to 93%. In 1987, the approximate cost of preventing one case of invasive cancer by an organised 3-yearly screening programme from age 20 to 65 years was estimated to be £13,000. Since about 50% of cases of invasive cervical cancer are curable, the cost of preventing one death would be £26,000. The diminishing return from shortening the screening interval suggests that if policy were to change from 3-yearly to 1-yearly, in England and Wales, 100 extra cases of invasive cancer would be prevented each year but the extra annual cost would be £110,000,000 — a marginal cost of £1,000,000 for each extra case prevented, or perhaps about £2,000,000 per extra death prevented. Compared with other returns for resources spent, such a policy change would be judged by most to have a very low priority.

General practitioners have a key role in the cervical cancer screening programme not merely by taking smears, but also in persuading reluctant patients to be screened, in ensuring that correct addresses are recorded on FHSA lists and in ensuring that women requiring further investigation are adequately followed up.

Breast cancer

There have been several prospective randomised controlled trials of screening for breast cancer, and a number of other evaluative studies. The screening method has always included X-ray mammography, supplemented in some cases by clinical examination of the breast. The first two trials, from New York[11] and from two Swedish countries,[12] each showed a statistically significant one-third reduction in mortality in a population who were offered screening compared with a control population. The reduction began to show two years after the introduction of screening and is still maintained — albeit at a slightly lower level — at follow-up to 18 years (New York) and 9 years (Sweden). Two further randomised trials and one prospective geographical comparison have since found lesser reductions (19%, 17% and 20%) in mortality which were not statistically significant. The relative protection apparently conferred by screening in three case-control studies is of the order of 50% to 65%. The current state of evidence from these various studies is well summarised by Forrest.[13] The prospective trial method is a true reflection of what will happen in practice in a population for whom a screening programme is provided as a public health service, but it tends to underestimate benefit to the screened individual because the study population includes non-attenders, and deaths among these must also be included in the comparison. Conversely, the case-control method overemphasises benefit to the individual because it compares risk of dying from the cancer in acceptors of screening with that in refusers, and the latter group tend to be at underlying higher risk.

All the breast screening trials have found that the reduction in mortality is concentrated in women aged over 50, when they were first invited to be screened, and there is no evidence at present that starting to screen women when they are under the age of 50 is of value. This may be at least partly because screening is less sensitive in premenopausal breasts. Another difficulty is that the death rate from breast cancer in young women is relatively low and none of the trials so far has had a sufficiently large sample of young women to give it statistical power to be confident of showing a difference. Further trials in young women are now in progress.

Similarly, there is no evidence that clinical examination of the breasts is effective as a screening test. It is much less sensitive than mammography, detecting only half to two-thirds of screen-detected cancers when both tests are used in combination. Conversely, mammography detects around 95% of screen-detected cancers. Another screening method whose value is unknown is breast self-examination. One study of districts in which every woman aged 45 to 64 was invited to a class to learn breast self-examination and provided with access to a clinic, compared subsequent breast cancer mortality with that in control districts with no such programme and found no difference.[14]

In the light of these findings, the UK breast screening programme is limited to 3-yearly mammography for women over 50, who are invited from general practitioners' registers to attend special screening centres. Even this level of screening is the subject of controversy because it is claimed that the reduction in risk of death which this may achieve is likely to be less than that shown in the early trials, and that the psychological morbidity induced by screening will be very great. However, studies of psychological morbidity in women attending for screening and in women with false positive screening results have been reassuring.[15] On the first occasion they are screened, up to 8% of women who turn out not to have cancer may be recalled for further investigation of a suspicious mammogram, falling to 3–4% at subsequent routine screens. The great majority of these false positive referrals can be confirmed as benign or normal by further mammograms and clinical examination, less than 1% requiring biopsy. The benign to malignant biopsy ratio is less than 1:1, the same as in unscreened women aged over 50 with symptomatic disease. However, just as the yield of cancer is greater than the incidence in unscreened women, so the prevalence of benign biopsies, particularly after the first screen, is also increased.

For women aged over 50 the reduction in risk of breast cancer death which is given by screening is felt by most to be worth the inconvenience and small risk of morbidity from a false positive referral. Given current levels of acceptance of screening and of sensitivity, it can be expected that between 1,000 and 1,500 breast cancer deaths could be prevented each year in the UK, once the programme has been fully implemented for over five years (which will be about the year 2000); the resource cost has been estimated as £3,500 per year of life gained (1987 prices).

Except in research trials, there is at present no case for screening symptomless women under the age of 50, no case for screening women of any age by clinical examination on its own, and no case for actively promulgating breast self-examination. However, women should be encouraged to report breast symptoms without delay and symptoms in women of any age should be thoroughly investigated. The value of screening women below 50 who have a strong family history of premenopausal breast cancer is unknown, but it seems reasonable to provide it for those women who request it.

Lung cancer

Three randomised controlled trials of screening for lung cancer have been published. The first, in London, randomised factories employing a total of 55,000 men aged 45 and over into a group offering 6-monthly chest X-rays for three years and group who were X-rayed only once at the end of the trial.[16] Although more resectable tumours were found in the screened group, there was no difference in the death rate from lung cancer between the two groups after three years. The second, Mayo clinic trial[17] screened 30,000 men and then randomised those in whom the findings had been negative into a group screened 4-monthly by chest X-ray and sputum cytology and a control group who were advised to have an annual chest X-ray. Again, more resectable tumours were found in the intensively screened group and their survival was better than that of control group cases, but after seven years there was no difference in lung cancer mortality between the two groups. The third, in Czechoslovakia,[18] had essentially similar results over a 6-year follow-up period.

A case-control study in East Germany found no relative protection against lung cancer deaths among subjects who had been screened. The prospective trials can be criticised on the grounds of lack of statistical power, contamination of the control group, and relatively short follow-up periods. Nevertheless the fact that their negative findings were substantiated by a case-control study (a method which tends to overestimate benefit) leads to the conclusion that screening is of little or no value. This adds extra weight to the urgency of primary prevention by curtailing cigarette smoking.

Testicular cancer

Concern about the increasing frequency of testicular cancer has led to pressure to promote testicular self-examination in young men. This form of screening has never been evaluated but, because chemotherapy now achieves cure rates of 90% or more, even in advanced cases, screening is probably unnecessary. Moreover, because there is no identifiable pre-invasive stage, screening can certainly not reduce incidence but might even increase it by overdiagnosis of borderline tumours. Thus screening for testicular cancer is not indicated.

Other cancer sites

Other tests available for cancer screening include the following: faecal occult blood for colorectal cancers and adenomas, ultrasound and CA 125 for ovarian cancer, barium X-ray for stomach cancer, mouth inspection for oral cancer, skin inspection for melanoma, urine cytology and haematuria tests for bladder cancer, rectal examination for prostate cancer, AFP for liver cancer, urinary vanillyl mandelic acid and homovanillic acid for neuroblastoma.

Trials are in progress for some of these, although even for the most intensively studied, colorectal cancer, it is still likely to be several years before a definitive answer is available. Without evidence of benefit there is no justification for offering these tests to symptomless people except within the context of an approved research study.

CONCLUSIONS AND RECOMMENDATIONS

1   **Cigarette smoking:** Up to 30% of all cancer deaths in the UK could be avoided if there were **no cigarette smoking**. During professional contacts with patients, and in advising the public at large, every opportunity should be taken by the medical profession to emphasise the risks of cigarette smoking. *Specific recommendations are given in Chapter 2.*

2   **Alcohol:** Similarly, in advising patients and others about the maximum 'safe' levels of alcohol consumption, doctors should emphasise that alcohol increases the risk of most cancers of the upper gastrointestinal and upper respiratory tracts, and that the

cancer risk is particularly important in those who smoke cigarettes. *Specific advice is given in Chapter 3.*

3   **Obesity:** Obesity increases the risks of cancer of the gall-bladder and endometrium.

4   **Diet:** It is sensible to eat plenty of fruit and green vegetables as these may help to reduce the risk of gastrointestinal and possibly other cancers. The addition of cereal fibre to the diet may also confer some protection against large bowel cancer. It should be made clear however that the link between these dietary constituents and cancer is not definitely proven and the level of protection they confer is unknown (*see Chapter 4*).

5   **Contraception:** Advice on which form of contraception couples should use entails weighing up the benefits and risks:

- Among the benefits, condoms protect against cervical and penile cancers; and long-term use of oral contraception protects against ovarian and endometrial cancers.

- Conversely, there may be an increased risk of breast cancer with prolonged use of oral contraception before the first pregnancy.

These benefits and risks are of course only a small part of the balance, in comparison with the immediate benefit of avoiding unwanted pregnancy and the risks of other diseases especially those of the cardiovascular and cerebrovascular systems.

6   **Hormone replacement therapy:** Women around the age of the menopause should be informed of the benefits and risks of hormone replacement therapy, the latter including a possible increased risk of breast cancer and a risk of endometrial cancer if unopposed oestrogen is given.

7   **Sunburn and melanoma:** Children should be protected against episodes of sunburn, by ensuring that they wear protective clothing such as hats and T-shirts and using sunscreen skin products especially before sunbathing. Similarly, fair-skinned people and those with multiple moles, should be advised against short-term bouts of exposure to the sun, such as occur during short holidays to hot sunny climates.

- People should be informed of the need to report changes in an existing mole or sudden growth of a new mole to their general practitioner without delay. General practitioners and other doctors should be aware of the danger signs of malignant melanoma and should make these priority referrals to a dermatologist.

8 **Environmental hazards:** Patients who enquire from their doctors about the risks of environmental carcinogens over which they have little or no personal control, such as radon gas, asbestos in buildings, or ionizing radiation around nuclear installations should be reassured that these risks are low (in the case of radon gas) or minute compared to those of smoking and other aspects of life-style. They should be referred for expert advice to their local Department of Public Health.

9 **Cervical screening:** General practitioners, family planning doctors, gynaecologists and genitourinary physicians should always ensure that they know the cervical screening history of all their adult women patients. Women who have not had a negative routine cervical smear within the previous five years should always be offered a screening test, and special care should be taken to ensure that those who have had a positive or suspicious smear are being followed up appropriately. Women who have had a negative routine smear within the previous three years should not be offered a further test, and requests for such testing should be answered with an explanation that it will confer virtually no extra protection, but will clog up the laboratory and thus may threaten facilities for screening other higher risk women.

10 **Breast screening:** General practitioners and other doctors consulted by women aged between 50 and 65 should enquire whether the woman has had a routine screening mammogram within the previous three years. If not, enquiry should be made as to whether she has yet been invited, and if not, she should be advised that, provided she is registered under her correct address with a general practitioner, she will be invited within the next 2–3 years. (All eligible women should have been invited at least once by the end of 1993.) If she has not attended for screening in response to an invitation she should be advised of the possible benefit to her of being screened, and the local breast screening office should be informed if she then agrees to be screened. Women aged over 65 should be informed that they can be screened on request at 3-yearly intervals, and should be told how to contact the local breast screening office. Women aged under 50 who request screening should be told that at their age its benefit is unproven.

11   **Screening for other forms of cancer:** People who enquire about screening for other forms of cancer should be told that its value is still uncertain, except for lung cancer where it is ineffective, and testicular cancer, where it is unnecessary.

12   **Inheritance risks:** There are a small number of families with an inherited risk of cancer and in whom the risk of cancer at a young age is particularly high, eg familial large bowel cancer, familial breast cancer, multiple endocrine neoplasia syndrome. Although of unproven value, screening may be offered to such families for reassurance.

7 Infectious disease

Prevention *vs* treatment

Infectious disease provides some of the best examples of the advantages of prevention over treatment. When antibiotics were developed and became widely used it was generally expected that infectious diseases would disappear. What was not appreciated was that although treatment would affect *mortality*, and also alter the course of a disease, including avoidance of complications and suffering, it would do little to prevent disease *morbidity*. The notification and death patterns for whooping cough, measles and diphtheria (Figs 7.1–7.3) show this well. Both measles and whooping cough were first made nationally notifiable in 1940. The number of deaths closely followed the pattern of notifications until the latter half of the 1940s when the numbers of deaths began to decrease but the number of cases notified did not. This suggests that more patients survived. In the late 1940s several developments could have accounted for this: the increasing use of antibiotic agents for the treatment of complications, better social conditions, including better nutrition, and possibly the introduction of the health service. These changes prevented deaths, but it was not until the introduction of vaccine that the incidence of infection appeared to have been altered.

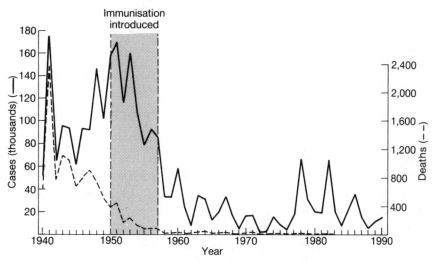

Fig. 7.1 *Whooping cough: notified cases and deaths in England and Wales, 1940–90.*
Source: *OPCS*.

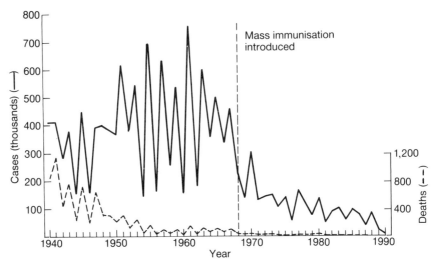

Fig. 7.2 *Measles: notified cases and deaths in England and Wales, 1940–90.* Source: *OPCS*.

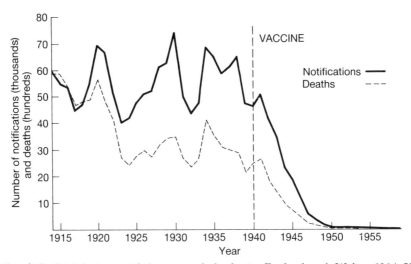

Fig. 7.3 *Diphtheria: notified cases and deaths in England and Wales, 1914–59.* Source: *OPCS*.

With diphtheria, however, the introduction of an effective vaccine, with the resultant decline in the number of cases, predated the health and social improvements mentioned above. Likewise, the number of deaths declined, but not because treatment improved—indeed the case-fatality ratio remained about the same throughout this period. These examples show that *primary prevention* is considerably more efficient and effective than other forms of prevention and treatment.

Throughout the 1950s and 1960s, the treatment of sexually transmitted

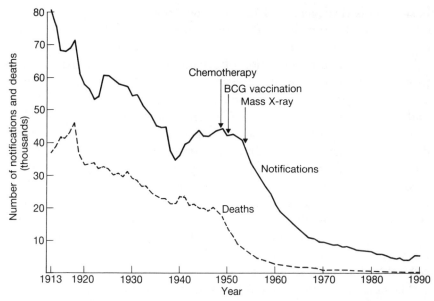

Fig. 7.4 *Respiratory tuberculosis: notified cases and deaths in England and Wales 1913–90.* Source: *OPCS.*

diseases (STDs)—especially gonorrhoea, syphilis and non-specific urethritis—improved considerably and mortality decreased dramatically, in spite of which there was an unprecedented rise in the incidence of these infections. The surge in the incidence of gonorrhoea and non-specific urethritis (NSU) was not matched by that of syphilis, probably because secondary prevention of syphilis was more successful. The influence of social trends on the spread of STDs is described later in this chapter.

In chronic infections such as tuberculosis where infectiousness persists or may increase as the disease progresses, treatment would be expected to contribute to prevention, and Fig. 7.4 shows that this may well have occurred. Nevertheless, the number of notified cases of tuberculosis had been decreasing for many years before the introduction of any medical intervention of proven efficacy. Other diseases, such as scarlet fever, have also declined without active medical intervention—curiously both in incidence and in severity.

The prevention of infectious disease is considered below under the headings Immunisation, Antibiotics, Physical Prevention of Spread, and Social and Organisational Factors.

Immunisation

Immunisation against infectious disease began with Jenner's work on vaccination as a method of protection against smallpox, but a rational basis for his discovery had to wait upon the work of Pasteur, three quarters of a century later. Pasteur promulgated the 'germ theory' of disease and showed, successively with chicken cholera, anthrax and rabies, that the administration of attenuated micro-organisms could protect against subsequent exposure to the wild agent. In the latter years of the 19th century, vaccination with killed typhoid organisms, and with diphtheria and tetanus toxoids was developed, and in this century successful vaccination against a larger number of important diseases has been achieved. Immunisation carried out on an immense scale has proved one of the most evidently successful agents of preventive medicine. During the last two decades, recombinant technology has been applied with great success to vaccine development, and new candidate vaccines, both against disease for which vaccines already exist, eg pertussis, and for other diseases for which vaccine control is not yet available, are being developed and promise even more efficient control with fewer disadvantages.[1]

The agents currently used are of several different types:

1. *Toxoids.* The component of the organism responsible for its pathogenic effect is altered in a way which removes toxicity while retaining immunogenicity, eg tetanus, diphtheria.

2. *Killed whole organisms.* Bacteria, eg *Bordella pertussis*, or viruses, eg inactivated poliomyelitis virus or yellow fever. The organism is killed in such a way that it retains its immunogenicity, but not its pathogenicity.

3. *Attenuated whole live organisms.* Virus vaccines, eg oral poliomyelitis, measles, mumps, rubella; bacterial vaccines eg BCG.

4. *Purified antigenic components of killed organisms.* For example, some influenza vaccines, hepatitis B surface antigen vaccine.

The effects of immunisation on the population at large are complex and depend on factors such as population size, the method and facility with which the organism disseminates, and the duration and degree of natural and vaccine-induced immunity. Vaccines against diseases which are communicable from person-to-person may induce some herd immunity, ie by reducing transmission rates they may produce a greater reduction in incidence than one would expect from the number vaccinated. In the case of a disease such as tetanus, caused by an organism widespread in cultivated soil, the aim of vaccination can only be to prevent disease in the individual vaccinated. Such vaccines cannot induce herd immunity. Likewise, there is no possibility of greatly influencing the infecting agent when a large reservoir of infection exists in inaccessible animal hosts, as with yellow fever.

By contrast, eradication is a possible aim when the organism is confined to the human host or has no animal or environmental reservoir and does not possess a capacity of latency and reactivation. Eradication has actually been achieved in the case of smallpox, and eradication of poliomyelitis is an aim of the World Health Organisation. Even for such a widespread disease as measles it is possible, by high and sustained immunisation, almost to achieve eradiction, although incomplete immunity from the few failures or partial failures of vaccine response may allow re-introduction of this highly-contagious virus to spread with ease even in a community with a generally high level of immunisation.[2]

Unwanted effects of vaccine

The problem of unwanted effects of vaccine is a major concern in immunisation programmes. Minor troubles, swelling and pain at the site of vaccination, and slight degrees of fever are common and rarely troublesome, but the same reactions sometimes occur in more serious form. Febrile convulsions occasionally ensue as a sequel to vaccination, since the current schedules of immunisation are carried out over an age span during which febrile convulsions are common. The vaccines currently in general use have a remarkably good safety record, but serious unwanted effects do occur, although rarely, and present a problem of increasing relative importance as the importance of the disease itself declines from the effect of the vaccination programme. Thus, the development of clinical poliomyelitis in approximately one in a million vaccine recipients or their contacts would appear of little significance in the presence of epidemic or endemic poliomyelitis. When, however, as in Britain today, no wild virus is normally circulating and in many years no poliomyelitis is reported, even a rare unwanted effect such as this presents in sharp relief.

The interplay between vaccine policy, public and professional attitudes and perceptions, and the possibility of important unwanted effects is well shown in the recent history of vaccination against pertussis. The publicity surrounding reports that whooping cough vaccine could cause brain damage in children led to a serious decline in immunisation rates. The subsequent epidemics of the disease demonstrated clearly, if in retrospect, both the good control which a relatively high level of vaccination had achieved, and also the prolonged unpleasantness and occasional dangers of the disease itself. It is now believed that serious neurological effects of pertussis vaccination, if they occur at all, are of great rarity and vastly exceeded in importance by the morbidity of the disease itself.

Current schedules of immunisation

The schedule of immunisation currently used in Great Britain (Table 7.1) aims to protect all children (other than those with genuine contra-indications to receiving a particular vaccine) against diphtheria, tetanus, pertussis, poliomyelitis, measles, mumps, rubella and tuberculosis. The actual schedule varies from time to time and is based on a pragmatic compromise between various, sometimes conflicting, factors such as the age at which the disease has its main impact, the age at which immune response is most favourable and the age at which children are most easily intercepted as their parents bring them to their general practitioner or child health clinics.[3]

Table 7.1   Schedule for routine immunisation

Age	Vaccine	Method of delivery
At 2 months At 3 months At 4 months	Diphtheria Whooping cough Tetanus	One injection (DPT)
	Polio	By mouth
At 12–18 months (usually before 15 months)	Measles Mumps Rubella	One injection (MMR)
3–5 years (around school entry)	Diphtheria Tetanus	Booster injection
	Polio	Booster by mouth
Girls 10–14 years	Rubella	One injection
Girls/boys 13 years	Tuberculosis	One injection (BCG)
School leavers	Tetanus	One injection
15–19 years	Polio	Booster by mouth

In addition, it is hoped to introduce vaccination against Haemophilus influenzae type b, an important cause of meningitis (and acute epiglottitis), in 1992, using one of the new conjugate vaccines which have already proved successful in clinical trials.

Vaccines not included in the routine schedule

Many other vaccines are available in addition to those in the routine schedule. Some of them are mainly relevant to travellers. They include active immunisation against typhoid, cholera, yellow fever, hepatitis B, rabies, some types of meningococci, and passive immunisation against hepatitis A. Others, however, are relevant to practice within the UK, although there is a good deal of controversy about the precise indications for some of them.

Influenza vaccine is recommended as an annual measure for those considered to be at special risk from this infection. These include people with chronic pulmonary, cardiac and renal disease; diabetes and those on immunosuppressive treatment.[3] Elderly people and children in residential homes and long-stay hospitals should also be given influenza vaccine.

The indications for *hepatitis B vaccine* are complex but include health care personnel and certain other occupational groups at risk of parenteral exposure, sexual partners of hepatitis B carriers, and post-exposure prophylaxis for infants born to mothers who are carriers.[4]

The role of vaccination against *pneumococcal disease*—for which a vaccine containing capsular polysaccharide from 23 serotypes is available—is accepted for some patients at particular risk, such as those with sickle cell disease or asplenia, but there is still controversy about how effective it would be if used on a larger scale,[5] for example, in the same population as that for which influenza vaccine is recommended.

WHO programme

On the world scale, plans have been dominated by the policies of the World Health Organisation which, in its *Extended Programme of Immunisation*, aims to immunise all the children in the world against six target diseases, diphtheria, tetanus, pertussis, poliomyelitis, measles and tuberculosis, with subsidiary national programmes against diseases of local importance, eg hepatitis B, rabies, Japanese encephalitis, depending on their importance in the particular country.

The availability of an effective, safe and cheap vaccine is insufficient to ensure a successful vaccine programme—achieving a high uptake in a population requires organisation, motivation (both political and professional) and health education.[6]

Prospects for new vaccines

The enormous impact of molecular biology on vaccine development has opened possibilities of great advance in vaccination.[7] Recombinant technology makes it possible to produce larger quantities of a desired antigen, when the whole organism may be difficult, dangerous or impossible to produce in amounts which can be used for vaccine production. One example already marketed and widely used is hepatitis B vaccine derived from hepatitis B surface antigen expressed in yeast cells and purified from them. Such antigens are entirely safe from the danger of infectivity, since they contain only the desired protective fraction of the genome of the causative virus, and not the infectious agent itself. Another use of 'genetic engineering' in vaccine production lies in the construction of attenuated organisms. Many of the present vaccines we have described are living attenuated forms of the organism concerned, eg measles virus vaccine and BCG (an altered form of the organism which causes bovine tuberculosis), and have proved safe and successful. It is now possible, however, to produce precisely targeted genetic attenuation in which, to give one example, the gene coding for the active subunit of cholera toxin is deleted from the bacterial genome. Recombinant methods can also be used to introduce genes which code for desired protective antigens into avirulent carrier organisms which can deliver the protective antigens to the reticulo-endothelial system. In theory at least, one delivery system, either as an injection, or a live oral vaccine, could be used to deliver a large number of antigens, making it possible to protect against many diseases with only two or three vaccine doses.

Although many of these advances are already in use in some human and veterinary vaccines, the process of vaccine development is long, difficult and expensive, involving both the costs of research and development and of the licensing procedures and clinical trials. Insurance against litigation related to possible vaccine damage has to be included and is responsible for almost the entire cost of pertussis vaccine in the USA (vaccine ca. 40 cents, insurance ca. 8 dollars). The consumer costs of many existing vaccines are far beyond the health budgets of many developing countries and the cost of testing and introducing new vaccines into the very communities most in the need of them presents formidable problems.

Passive immunisation

All the vaccines in widespread use for the protection of communities depend on active immunisation, a process whereby the immune system is stimulated by the vaccine in such a way as to simulate natural immunity, so that a rapid and protective response is evoked when the subject encounters the naturally occurring pathogen. Passive immunisation, in which antibody, usually of human origin, is injected to confer protection, is of much more limited scope since the injected antibody has a relatively short duration of action (the half-life of human IgG is about four weeks). Nevertheless passive immunisation does have a limited role in prophylaxis.[8] Its main use in otherwise healthy people is to confer temporary—and incomplete—protection against hepatitis A infection for travellers to the many areas of high prevalence of this virus. Of great importance are the preparations of human immunoglobin with high levels of antibody against particular antigens. The use of human anti-tetanus immune globulin is widespread in A & E departments for patients with high tetanus-risk wounds. Patients with some haematological malignancies or on immunosuppressive drugs receive anti-varicella immune globulin when in contact with chickenpox because of the grave threat this infection presents to them, and infants born to mothers with acute or chronic hepatitis B infection receive anti-hepatitis B immune globulin in addition to active immunisation with hepatitis B vaccine, as do those in accidental contact with material contaminated with blood containing hepatitis B virus.[8]

Antibiotics in prevention

The main role of antibiotics, and an important one, is in the treatment of established infection, and their beneficial influence here has been enormous.

It is nevertheless true that the morbidity and mortality attributable to many important pathogens had been declining before the era of antibiotics and continued to decline following their introduction; it seems certain that important changes have taken place in the pathogenic potential of many important organisms, probably often as a result both of changing virulence of the parasite and changing susceptibility of the host. Thus, in the early years of this century scarlet fever remained a serious disease carrying a substantial mortality, whereas now its effects are usually no more serious than that of a streptococcal throat infection without the rash. So that, while in some infections the beneficial effects of antibiotics are well established and evident, for example in bacterial meningitis, bacterial pneumonia and septicaemia, in milder illnesses their proper role is hard to establish.

In preventive medicine, antibiotics have certain limited but well-defined roles. These fall into two main categories: the prevention of specific infections and the prevention of infection following surgery.

Prevention of specific infections

Antibiotic and chemoprophylactic agents may be used to prevent specific infections from which a subject may be at risk because of individual special susceptibility to the pathogen or because of a particular danger of exposure. Some examples of the use of these agents in this context are illustrated in Table 7.2.

Prevention of infection following surgery

A second type of chemoprophylaxis, with more widespread application, is concerned with the prevention of infection following surgery. The concept that infection associated with surgery might be diminished by the use of antibiotics seems at first sight a reasonable one, but earlier attempts to achieve this kind of preventive intervention were ineffective or even harmful; infection rates were not lessened, even increased, and the widespread use of antibiotics in hospital for ineffective attempts at chemoprophylaxis led to the emergence of antibiotic-resistant strains of bacteria as a major cause of hospital infection. During the 1980s, however, a much sounder and possibly economically efficient basis for surgical prophylaxis was established, and the effect of modern methods of chemoprophylaxis in reducing rates of infection in several forms of surgery has now been fully established by controlled trials.[9] Antibiotic

Table 7.2 Some examples of chemoprophylactic agents used in the prevention of infection

Disease/pathogen	Subject	Agent used
Meningococcus	Close contact	Rifampicin, others
Malaria	Traveller	Chloroquine, proguanil, others
Tuberculosis	Newborn contact	Isoniazid
Subacute bacterial endocarditis	Rheumatic heart disease (and congenital heart disease)	Penicillin, amoxycillin, others
Strep. pneumoniae	Sickle cell disease/ splenectomy	Penicillin
Pneumocystis carinii	HIV disease	Co-trimoxazole, pentamidine

These types of agents may be of some importance in communicable disease control, for example, in the control of outbreaks of meningococcal disease, but are commonly restricted in their application to relatively uncommon situations of restricted groups of subjects.

prophylaxis is of particular value in relation to operations involving normally highly contaminated surfaces, eg lower bowel surgery, which carry a very high risk of infective complications. By contrast, antibiotics are not given in 'clean' surgical operations, with the important exception of major surgery involving insertion of prostheses, eg heart valve surgery or hip replacement. Although infection is rare in this type of surgical procedure, when it does occur its consequences may be extremely serious.

The principles of chemoprophylaxis now established in relation to surgery involve the use of only very short courses of the appropriate antibiotic, varying between a single dose and a course lasting no more than 24 or 48 hours, and beginning immediately before operation, usually at the time of induction of anaesthesia, with the aim of achieving adequate concentrations of the antibacterial agent within the wound during the course of the operation and for a short time after it. The efficacy of such methods is well established and it is hoped that their application as a component of an agreed hospital antibiotic policy will minimise disturbance of the patient's indigenous flora and thus diminish the spread of resistant hospital flora. This type of restrictive antibiotic policy also leads to potential economies in the hospital drug budget, since the use of antibiotics for attempted prophylaxis accounted, in recent years, for about 30% of the total drug budget in many American hospitals.

Physical methods for the prevention of spread of infection

Body protection

Physical methods of preventing infective organisms from entering the body have a limited role to play in preventing infection. Organisms can enter the body through the skin, mucous membranes (including those of the genital tract), conjunctiva, respiratory tract, the gastrointestinal tract and transplacentally.

Protection of areas of skin exposed to penetrative organisms such as leptospires, ancylostomes and schistosomes may be difficult when the whole body is exposed, eg swimming in contaminated waters. Vigorous towelling after exposure to schistosome contaminated waters is said to reduce risk. Most of the organisms causing sexually transmitted infections probably penetrate intact mucous membrane. Condoms are advocated for prevention of sexually transmitted diseases but compliance is usually poor, particularly among those who are most at risk. The conjunctival route of infection can theoretically be avoided by wearing goggles but this is clearly impractical in most situations. Fatal laboratory infections such as rabies acquired conjunctivally can be avoided by following approved laboratory safety measures. Similarly the wearing of masks to avoid acquiring infection by the respiratory route is not feasible except in special instances.

Prevention of infection in hospitals

It has long been recognised that hospitals, intended as they are to heal the sick, may also place them at risk of infection. The work of Holmes and of Semmelweiss on the spread of puerperal sepsis by doctors, and Lister's discoveries leading to improved control of surgical sepsis, were among the most important medical advances in the 19th century. Unfortunately, although an enormous body of knowledge is now available about the causes and control of hospital infection, the problem is still a large one, partly because of the medical advances which have improved the outlook for many patients with serious defects of their immune mechanisms. In particular, areas of a modern hospital such as intensive care units, neonatal units and units for the treatment of haematological malignancy treat vulnerable patients in circumstances prone to the selection of dangerous—and often antibiotic-resistant— pathogens. Nor is the problem of hospital infection confined to these special areas. A survey of 18,000 patients in acute units in 43 hospitals in the UK showed that 19.1% of them had infections, and that half of these (9.2%) had been acquired in hospital.[10] The most common types of hospital infection are of the urinary tract, wounds, lower respiratory tract, and skin. Hospital-acquired infections vary from the trivial, through to those causing delay in hospital discharge, to life-threatening conditions such as septicaemia and bacterial shock syndrome.

The long period of seeming indifference to hospital infection, fostered as it was by over-optimism about the control of infection in general, has fortunately come to an end, and there is much concern that hospitals can be dangerous to those who enter them. The prevention and control of hospital infection is a large subject, far beyond the scope of this report but its principles can be summarised. Control is based on:

- careful training in good hygienic practice (doctors are notable for their poor hand-washing techniques),
- use of suitable isolation procedures when necessary,
- good practice in sterilisation, disinfection, cleaning and waste disposal,
- the establishment of infection control policies for the hospital as a whole and for units of special importance within it such as operating theatres.

Isolation facilities should include provision of a sufficient number of single rooms and preferably an isolation unit in which a high level of practice in infectious disease control can be fostered and maintained.

It is evident that the problem of hospital infection affects many areas of hospital life, and organisational structures are needed to plan and implement control policies. *Infection control nurses* now play an important part in this work, spanning as they do the gap between infection control committee and the microbiology laboratory on the one hand, and the wards and theatres on the other. Hospital infection control policies are suitable for monitoring by medical audit. It is also necessary to provide for urgent intervention by pre-arranged procedures in the event of an outbreak of any unusual or unexpected infection.

Antibiotics have a limited but definite role in the prevention of hospital infection, and this is discussed on p 100.

This section has been concerned with infection in hospitals, but *schools* and *day care facilities for children* are also important focal points in the spread of infection, and hygienic standards need to be carefully maintained.

Environment

Measures aimed at altering some factor or factors in the environment have been used, sometimes effectively, for many centuries before the 'germ theory' of infectious diseases was developed.

Water   Sanitation and water purification have been particularly effective in prevention of infection. Water can be extremely efficient in spreading gastrointestinal and other infections and faecal contamination from animals and humans is common, especially with surface waters. Although several vaccines can be combined for ease of administration, vaccines are disease-specific in their protective effects, whereas treatment of water prevents a large number of different infections—viral, bacterial and protozoal—which only have in common that they are spread by the faecal-oral route. They include typhoid and cholera, viral hepatitis types A and E, *Giardia lamblia* and cryptosporidiosis.

Sanitation is the safe disposal and treatment of faeces and urine. An efficient sewage system is usually necessary. Sewage treatment works render the sewage microbiologically harmless. The disposal of raw sewage to natural waters such as lakes, rivers and seas is hygienically, aesthetically and environmentally undesirable and there is suspicion that bathing in these waters may cause illness.

The recognition that serious infection can be caused by inhaling aerosols from water contaminated by *Legionella pneumophila*—through jacuzzis, cooling towers and showers—has meant that it is not always adequate to treat water meant only for drinking, and the avoidance of legionellosis acquired from industrial and other buildings requires guidelines based on regular and adequate maintenance of air conditioning and plumbing systems.[11]

The chemical contamination of drinking water, for example by aluminium or lead, cannot be removed by ordinary filtration or chlorination, and vigilance and care are required to prevent incidents of contamination. Some hazards in water, such as blue-green algae and red tide, are caused by natural phenomena.

Vectors of infection   The transmission of many diseases of overwhelming world importance, such as malaria, filariasis, trypanosomiasis, leishmaniasis and arbovirus infections, is mediated through arthropod vectors. With the exception of Lyme disease, vector-borne diseases have little relevance to disease in the UK except to contribute to the toll of illness in returning travellers, although a few cases of malaria have arisen through transmission in warm weather by mosquitos arriving in planes ('airport malaria').

Mechanical transmission of infection by contamination of flies makes a contribution to the faecal-oral spread of infection, and control of insects is a necessary component of any food hygiene programme.

Pets   Some of man's best friends may reward him with an unpleasant illness. Psittacosis may be acquired from birds, and imported birds are quarantined and treated. The sexual cycle of toxoplasma takes place in the cat intestine; human infection probably mostly follows ingestion of food contaminated by oocysts. Rabies is prevented in this country by restriction of importation of animals, although a vaccine is also available. Strict hygiene is most important when handling animals and pets, and animal bites require careful attention since several potentially dangerous infections can be transmitted by them.

Travel   Travel may present special risks. Immunisation is only effective for a small number of conditions (see page 93), and care with food and water is important. Traveller's diarrhoea is a serious problem in some countries, with attack rates occasionally reaching 80%, and is difficult to prevent. The increasing prevalence of drug-resistant malaria also presents a serious problem, and in many parts of the world physical methods of protection (mosquito nets, repellants and protective clothing) have again become the most valuable preventive measures.[12]

Food

Notified cases of food poisoning have shown a sharp increase recently (Fig. 7.5). The prevention of food poisoning is a complex subject which involves the producer, the food processor or manufacturer, the retailer, the restaurateur and the consumer.

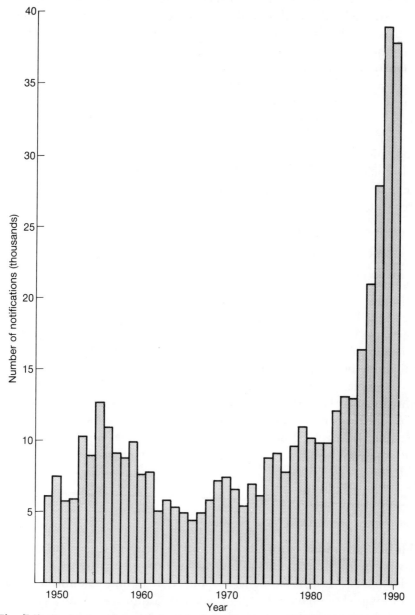

Fig. 7.5 *Food poisoning: annual notifications, England and Wales, 1949–90.* Source: *OPCS.*

Food of animal origin may be contaminated because of infection in the animal, eg salmonella in eggs or chickens, or because of 'natural' organisms in the animal, eg *Clostridium perfringens* in meat.[13] Food poisoning from this source is usually avoidable by thorough cooking and correct handling of food.

Certain toxic biochemical substances present naturally in food can be destroyed only by thorough cooking, eg red kidney beans; others, such as solanines in green potatoes, may be avoided by correct growing and storage of potatoes.

Dried, imported foods may also be contaminated, presumably during the drying process, eg salmonellas in desiccated coconut or peppercorns. Adequate quality control of imported sources of food is an important means of prevention but is difficult and expensive to achieve. It is however the only way of avoiding food poisoning from ready-to-eat foods such as chocolate.[14]

In the home and restaurant kitchen, food hygiene remains the main method of prevention of food poisoning. Common faults in food preparation[13] are:

- cross-contamination from raw to cooked food,
- extended storage of food at too warm a temperature, and
- inadequate reheating or thawing.

In the retailer's shop, inadequate separation of raw and cooked foods (eg cooked next to raw chicken in butcher's shops) is a common fault. The most obvious way of preventing these faults in food preparation is by improving public knowledge of food hygiene. Although much remains to be done in this field, there have been some notable successes, for example the large outbreaks of salmonella food poisoning from Christmas turkeys experienced in the early 1970s are now rare, as most caterers and housewives are aware of the dangers of inadequate thawing and cooking of turkey. Adequate training of caterers should go some way towards ensuring safer food in restaurants and catered functions.

Problems of prevention of food poisoning

Whilst precautions outlined above will prevent most food poisoning, its prevention is becoming an increasingly complex problem.

Foodborne *Listeria monocytogenes* infection is one example of food poisoning which may need additional precautions, such as storage of food below 4 degrees C for no longer than about 48 hours. Contamination of the inside of a hen's egg with salmonella as occurred in the recent outbreak of salmonellosis, has created particular problems because eggs are often eaten raw or lightly cooked. This has meant that prevention needs to be aimed at a very early stage, during the process of husbandry, and this type of problem is proving much more difficult to control.

Food manufacturing processes are on the whole extremely safe, with many reputable manufacturers using the HACCP system (Hazard Analysis and Critical Control Point system) to ensure food safety. Nevertheless, contamination does occur from time to time and recent examples in the UK have included chocolate and powdered infant milk.[14,15] Even minimal contamination of widely distributed foods can cause large outbreaks of food poisoning, and such outbreaks, together with the problems of salmonella contamination of eggs and listeria were the stimulus for the formation of the Richmond Committee to study this. The large number of recommendations in their report[16] illustrate the complex nature of the control of food poisoning. They include recommendations for a nationwide system for the microbiological surveillance and assessment of food, and pay special attention to monitoring contamination in the poultry food processing industry. Other recommendations include the need for further research on the impact of infectious intestinal disease in general practice and on the problem of listeriosis, the need for better liaison and information systems between veterinary and medical sources, and the need for training in outbreak control.

Bovine spongiform encephalopathy

Much has also been made by the public of the risk to humans from eating meat and offal from cows infected with bovine spongiform encephalopathy. There is no evidence as yet that human infection can occur from this source, but the outbreak in cattle could almost certainly have been avoided by using heat rather than chemical rendering of animal waste for feeding to cows.[17]

Organisational and social aspects of prevention of infection

Organisational aspects

The organisation of preventive health services plays an important part in preventing infectious disease. An efficient administration is crucial to a high vaccine uptake rate in a community. A relevant *surveillance–notification system*, characterised by timeliness, completeness of reporting, and accompanied by prompt intervention where necessary, whether at local or national levels, is of proven value.[18] A surveillance system ensures that outbreaks are recognised early, for investigation and control, or for tracing and treatment of contacts of individual cases. Quarantine is now rarely used except with imported animals. A national unit for the surveillance of infection and investigation of outbreaks has also proved valuable in those countries which have one, because such a unit acts as a central source of information for early warning and control, as a co-ordinating centre, and as a national training centre.

Laws for the control of infection, used judiciously, are essential. Those relating to water safety and to food handling and distribution are especially important. The muzzling of dogs was essential in the control of rabies in England, and the importation and quarantine laws are undoubtedly a worthwhile safeguard. Byelaws for the compulsory registration of cosmetic skin piercing (tattooing, ear piercing) and acupuncture enabled guidelines for hygiene to be enforced and have probably helped to prevent hepatitis B and AIDS from being transmitted in this way. The notification system requires the statutory reporting of certain infections, although the legal powers, either to prosecute for failure to notify or for the control of infection, are seldom used.

Health education plays some part in the prevention of infection, as shown by the example given about defrosting and cooking Christmas turkeys. Education plays a part in improving the uptake of vaccines, although it often needs to be directed more at the health personnel involved with the administration of the vaccine than at those who are to be vaccinated. Education also plays a part in avoiding many travel-associated infections.

Social aspects

Many infections, in common with other diseases, have a close association with social trends. These include the sexually-transmitted diseases (STDs) including AIDS, which clearly are related to sexual attitudes and behaviour, and infection transmitted by intravenous drug addiction. Infections influenced by social attitudes can be extremely difficult to control and the availability of effective treatment may have some serious side-effects on public health. For example, the increasing availability of effective, cheap, safe and easy to administer antibiotics since the 1960s may have contributed to the increase in STDs, as has the contraceptive pill. This means that the sexually-transmitted diseases are difficult to prevent and control. Paradoxically, however, the arrival of the AIDS epidemic, itself stimulated by social and other factors, in turn appeared to have temporarily stemmed the rise in STDs. Education may produce some return with intravenous drug addiction, as may a needle-exchange scheme, but prevention clearly needs to be directed at more fundamental questions such as why people need to abuse drugs, as well as to effective policing of drug pushers and drug availability. Clearly, prevention of drug abuse and the control in general of diseases influenced by social fashion are relatively ineffective at present, and there must remain some pessimism for the future.

Social and economic factors are also associated with many other infections, for example respiratory infections are associated with poor housing, and high immunisation rates are more difficult to achieve in highly mobile and disadvantaged populations. The relationships between social factors and childhood infections are further discussed in Chapter 10.

CONCLUSIONS AND RECOMMENDATIONS

1 Immunisation against infectious disease is a highly effective form of preventive medicine. Health workers can improve vaccine uptake by efficient conduct of immunisation programmes and by taking part in health education activities concerned with immunisation.

2 Antibiotics have a limited role in the prevention of infection both in hospital and in the community. Good antibiotic practice may help to limit the spread of antibiotic resistance which has imposed serious restrictions on the use of many previously valuable agents.

3 Good hospital practice must involve sound methods for infection control and the budgetary provisions to implement and monitor them.

4 Reliable and up-to-date advice about prevention of infection (and other hazards) should be readily available to prospective travellers.

5 The control of water and food-borne diseases requires a combination of research input, the creation of good codes of practice in farming, food manufacture, catering and building engineering, and widespread health education endeavours. Some ultimate legal sanctions are also essential.

8 Accidents

Introduction

Throughout history accidents of one form or another have been responsible for death and disability on a massive scale. Archaeological evidence shows clear evidence of trauma. Primitive man was always facing hazards from the wild animals he hunted, from rivers and the sea, from his enemies and even from domestic chores. Modern man still has not mastered the hazards of his own inventions. The quest for excitement and adventure, the fiercely competitive nature of many activities and the hazards built into man's environment all add up to considerable everyday risk.

A report of the Royal College of Surgeons[1] states:

> Injury from whatever source is a leading cause of long and short-term disability, yet it is paradoxical that our present age seems intent on discovering more sophisticated means of producing injury whilst at the same time developing more expert ways of salvaging victims of accidents.

Whilst there must eventually be an element of risk-taking in all human activities, the emphasis of accident prevention efforts must be to encourage 'sensible' precautions whenever possible, without detracting from the enjoyment or quality of life.

There is much that can be done to reduce accidents including improvements in the environment, education and legislation. However, human behaviour can contribute most to accident prevention, and it may be here that health staff can make a contribution to changing attitudes and awareness, modifying behaviour and thus to achieving a real reduction in accidents.

Epidemiology

The size of the problem

Accidents are the biggest killer and a major cause of disability in the age group 1–35 in the United Kingdom (Fig. 1.1, 1.2). For one-half of the lifespan for males and one-third for females the biggest hazard to life is from an accident.

Whilst injury and poisoning (excluding suicide) do not figure prominently in the total number of deaths in England and Wales (2.4% in 1989), they do account for a significant loss of life and loss of productive years of life because the majority of accidental deaths occur at a young age.

Accidents by age and sex

The patterns of accidents vary considerably in different age and sex groups. Young children and older people tend to experience accidents mainly related to their home environment. Older children and young adults experience a different group of accidents due to their more wide ranging activities.

The Office of Population Censuses and Surveys (OPCS) death returns[2] divide accidents into:

  i transport,

 ii home, and

iii 'elsewhere'.

Transport accidents cover mainly motor vehicle road accidents, whilst 'elsewhere' includes both work and sport and leisure accidents. Other sources of information on deaths include the Department of Transport[5] and the Health and Safety Commission. The latter has collected details of both deaths and non-fatal injuries at work since 1981. The recording and provision of accurate worthwhile information on hospital admissions and attendances due to accidents remains fragmentary and rudimentary. Only a few specialised studies provide information on disability following accidents.

For most people the actual risk of having an accident is greatest of all in the home because most people spend most of their time there. The greatest risk for death and serious injury is on the road. Most accidents at work, sport and leisure are a relatively low risk except for well-recognised high risk occupations like construction and deep sea fishing. The most hazardous sporting activities include horse riding, air sports, motor sports and mountaineering.

Accidents in children (0–14 years)

After the age of one year, accidents are the most important cause of death in children and result in about 10,000 children becoming permanently disabled each year. The overall accident experience of children is shown in Fig. 8.1. The major causes of death are road traffic accidents, fire, suffocation, drowning and poisoning. By far the most important cause is road traffic accidents with 40% of the total accidental deaths in childhood.

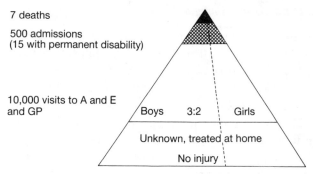

Fig. 8.1 *Injury experience of children in a typical health district in one year for a population of 250,000 of which 50,000 were children.* Source: *Ref. 6.*

There are marked differences in the accident experience of children by age as well as by sex. Babies under one year generally experience fewer accidents and these are nearly always at home. Toddlers also experience their accidents mainly in the home but they are beginning to explore their environment more widely and may come to grief outside. By the time they are four or five years old children have fewer accidents at home and more at school, at sport and especially at play. Road traffic accidents become more important as the child gets older.

An important factor in all accidents, but especially those of children, is a marked social class difference that is far greater for accidents than for all other forms of illness in childhood (Fig. 8.2). There is also a considerable 'grey area' of carelessness and neglect between obvious child abuse (non-accidental injury) and genuine accidents. A healthy alertness by health staff will help to differentiate in the majority of cases.

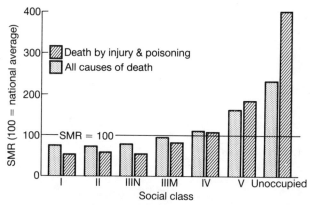

Fig. 8.2 *Standardised mortality ratios (SMRs) for children (aged 1–15 years), by social class, England and Wales, 1979–80, 82–83.* Source: *OPCS.*

Accidents in teenagers and young adults (15–35 years)

This is the age group with the highest proportion of total deaths due to accidents. More than two-thirds of all the teenage (15–19) and young adult (20–24) male deaths and nearly one-half of the female deaths in this age group are the result of accidents. The major cause by far is road traffic accidents (RTAs) with nearly half of the males dying from this cause. The next major cause is poisoning, mainly suicides.

The non-fatal accidents experienced by the 15–34 age group are RTAs, sporting and recreational accidents and, to a much lesser extent, assault and accidents at work. Many of these accidents, especially in the male, are due to bravado, recklessness and inexperience; alcohol plays a significant part in many of them (see Chapter 3). Drugs, including prescribed drugs, and solvents play a lesser role being involved in fewer than 5% of accidents in this group.

Accidents in middle aged adults (35–64 years)

The relative importance of accidents as a contribution to all deaths rapidly falls from age 35 (Fig. 1.1). The actual death rate still shows a slight rise with increasing age from 35 onwards in females and 55 onwards in males (Fig. 8.3). The gap between males and females also steadily falls with increasing age. Road traffic accidents continue to play an important role in accidental death in 35–64 year olds, and are responsible for almost one-quarter of all the accidental deaths in both males and females.

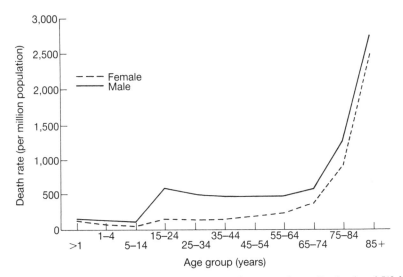

Fig. 8.3 *Death rates due to injury and poisoning by age and sex, England and Wales, 1989.* Source: *OPCS.*

Poisonings assume an even greater significance in this group with 1 in 5 of the male and 2 in 5 of the female accidental deaths from this cause. The majority of these come into the self-inflicted (suicide) class with some also due to homicide. Although suicide is not really an accident it is included in the broad classification of accidents in the International Classification of Diseases. Many suicides may be considered to be accidental because the person did not intend to take his or her life but was making a 'call for help'.

The non-fatal accidents of middle-aged adults derive mainly from RTAs, sport, recreation and the home. Activities such as 'DIY' and gardening become an increasing source of accidents. Alcohol is probably contributory in at least 1 in 5 of all the accidents in this age group.

Accidents in older people (65 years and over) (see also Chapter 11)

Fracture of the femur has been steadily increasing in the elderly in both numbers and rates in recent years.[3] Falls are responsible for over 60% of the female accidental deaths over 75 and over 40% of the male accidental deaths in this age group. Road traffic accidents account for 20% of accidental deaths in males over 75 and just over 10% of the female deaths. Well over 85% of all the RTA fatalities in the elderly are in pedestrians, and are often due to confusion with traffic and poor eyesight.[4]

Falls in the elderly often occur spontaneously. On other occasions they are the result of tripping over carpets or wiring in the house or loose pavements or ice in the street. There is frequently a background of postural hypotension, cardiac arrhythmia or medication or a combination of these. Older people who fall have often been very immobile and frequently have substantial osteoporosis. The problem is discussed in more detail in Chapter 11.

The elderly also come to grief by burns often due to carelessness with cigarettes, open fires or cooking fires. Poisoning may be due to confusion with drugs or due to deliberate overdosage. A small proportion of the deaths in the elderly are due to alcohol including some of those on the road and by drowning.

Death by accident only accounts for a very small proportion of the total deaths in the elderly. The death rate from accidents however is still considerably greater in the over 75s than in any other age group (Fig. 8.3).

Trends in accidents

There has been a steady decline in death rates due to accidents in Britain ever since the regular recording of deaths in the 1850s. One

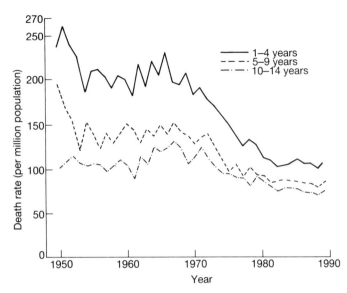

Fig. 8.4 *Trends in death rates due to childhood accidents. England and Wales, 1950–89.* Source: *Ref. 6.*

surprise is that, even with the ever-increasing volume of traffic, death rates from road traffic accidents continue to fall.[5]

Trends over the last 40 years in accidental deaths in childhood are shown in Fig. 8.4. The steady decline from the mid 1960s was due to a marked decline in deaths due to poisoning, notably in the 1–4 year old age group resulting from use of childproof containers, but also due to improvements in other areas like road traffic accidents, drowning and suffocation.[6]

Accidental deaths for all ages show falls in the last decade for both sexes (Fig. 8.5), but with the rate for females falling faster than that for males.

International comparisons

Comparison with other countries is often made difficult by different standards of recording and classification. In spite of this the World Health Organisation publishes regular returns of deaths by cause for many countries.

When comparisons are made of death rates for accidents, the UK compares very favourably with nearly all countries. For many years the UK had one of the lowest (if not the lowest) death rates for accidents and it is only recently that the Scandinavian countries, especially Sweden, have reached similar low levels. One anomaly is in

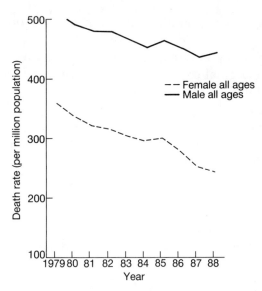

Fig. 8.5 *Death rates due to injury and poisoning, England and Wales, 1979–88.* Source: *OPCS.*

pedestrian deaths where the UK death rate, especially for children, is substantially higher than that in most European countries.

Measures for accident prevention

Accidents and their resulting trauma are different from many other diseases in that their cause is invariably known. Their prevention is, in theory, always possible. The reality is very different. Accidents happen 'even in the best regulated circles' and will go on happening. In young people they may be seen as a form of learning experience. One of the strong motivations in accident prevention must be to reduce severity. A series of trivial accidents may be quite acceptable but the more serious ones are not.

The standard measures used for the prevention of accidents may be classified for simplicity into: environment, enforcement and education.

Environment

Most of the hazards of the natural environment such as those caused by the sea or the weather are beyond man's control, and where the natural environment can be modified, for example by deforestation, the effects are often adverse.

Elements of the man-made environment also present dangers; for example, road systems, housing and even playgrounds and leisure facilities are all sites of accidents, as are places of work see Chapter 9). Although making the built environment safer may be costly, overall this may be a marginal cost. When it is known that accidents can be prevented by building in safety measures at source, such measures should always be incorporated into the design and structure.

Accident prevention should be looked at as an environmental issue. Much can be done—from improving streets and developing safer cars to improving the design and building of houses.

Enforcement

Legislation is sometimes necessary to reduce accidents. Examples of such legislation are the large number of laws and regulations that apply to motoring where there is need to have control of vehicle standards, speed limits and behaviour on the road.

Education

In an ideal world both general and specific education would ensure that people of all ages would be fully equipped with the information and the skills to avoid the majority of accidents. In practice, this ideal is far from being achieved and there is much scope for improved training of the public in accident prevention. In spite of the many daily hazards they encounter, there is a great deal that people can do to help themselves. Pedestrians, for example, can make themselves more conspicuous to traffic. Appropriate safety or protection devices can reduce the severity of injury: the use of protective clothing at work, seat belts in cars, and helmets for riders of motorcycles, bicycles and horses are examples of devices that can markedly reduce injury. It is regrettable that people are often unwilling to take a proven and reliable precaution. The wearing of cycle helmets in Britain is a good case in point: five years ago only 1% of cyclists wore helmets and even now (1991) fewer than 5% wear them, although use is much greater in university towns. Many horseriders have now accepted the message and those under 14 years are now required by law to wear approved helmets on the road. However, some riders well-known to the public are still frequently seen (and photographed) without helmets.

It is often considered unfashionable or 'cissy' to take too much notice of safety precautions. The 'risk compensation' theory suggests that even if notice is taken of one safety measure, risk may be transferred to another activity. An often quoted example is the aggressive driver who behaves even more recklessly when forced to wear a seat belt.

How can health staff help?

Doctors and health professionals are in a unique position to do a great deal for the prevention of accidents. They have easy access to information on the causes and consequences of accidents and can comment with authority on where and how efforts at accident prevention should be directed. Directors of public health are now required to produce an annual report on the state of health in their districts, so that a commentary on the effects of accidents in the community, the means taken to combat them and some evaluation of the intervention measures can be expected.[8]

Doctors and health staff have often been helpful in educational activities, in changing the man-made environment and in helping to

Table 8.1   Accident prevention measures which may be carried out by doctors and health staff

- General education of patients (eg on fire safety, children in cars, avoiding falls, use of cycle helmets, disposal of unused medicines)
- Opportunistic education of patients on a specific issue when the occasion arises (eg on the storage of medicines during a home visit)
- Detailed enquiry into the cause of individual accidents and advice on prevention of future accidents
- Observance of great care when prescribing any drugs which may increase accident potential, especially in the elderly and in those driving or using machinery (eg psychotropic drugs, tranquillisers, antidepressants) (British Medical Association[9])
- Thorough medical examinations and provision of advice (eg for insurance, for those who are over 70, post-coronary, epilepsy, and stroke) (Medical Commission on Accident Prevention, 1985[10])
- Provision of specific advice to patients known to be at risk (eg on head protection, sporting equipment)
- Checking and advising of hazards in the home, especially for the very young and very old (eg stairs, kettles, medicine storage, household chemicals, electricity, DIY equipment, window latches, baby walkers)
- Display of accident prevention and safety material in surgeries, clinics and public areas including waiting areas in outpatients and A&E departments (eg on drinking and driving; children in cars etc)
- Adequate screening for employment (eg HGV drivers)
- Provision of advice or teaching (eg on first-aid and resuscitation) and encouragement of correct training and coaching techniques for sports and leisure activities

frame laws. For example doctors provided evidence of the value of seat belts, helped in the design, persuaded people to use them and campaigned for changes in the law to make their use mandatory. There are many other examples in home safety, work safety and in sport and leisure where the direct action of doctors has brought about change.

Doctors can also influence accident prevention by advising individual patients about avoidable dangers in their environment and counselling them to alter risk behaviour.

Although not strictly accident prevention, another way in which health staff contribute to preventing morbidity from accidents is by first-aid and resuscitation for accident victims. There is still much scope for improved first-aid training both for the public (in Scandinavian countries all children are taught emergency aid and survival) and for doctors in particular.

Summaries of accident prevention measures that may be introduced during contacts between individual patients and doctors and health staff are shown in Table 8.1.

CONCLUSIONS AND RECOMMENDATIONS

1   Accidents are responsible for just over 2% of deaths in the UK. Within the age group 1–35 years they are the major killer and a major cause of disability. All accidents are, in theory, preventable, but in reality accidents will continue to occur. One of the overall objectives of accident prevention work must be to reduce death and serious injury.

2   Good progress has been made in accident prevention in the United Kingdom but a number of specific problems require further attention. These include:

   • Pedestrian road traffic accidents;
   • Burns and scalds in children;
   • Car occupant and motorcycle accidents in teenagers and young people;
   • Work, sport and leisure accidents;
   • All forms of home accidents, especially falls in the elderly.

   Alcohol is a contributory factor in around 20–30% of all accidents.

3   There is still scope to reduce accidents by improvements in the environment and changes in legislation. In the end however, it is changes in attitude and behaviour that will bring accident and injury experience down to acceptable levels.

4   Health staff can make an important contribution to accident prevention by counselling and advising patients.

Appendix
Sources of useful information on accident prevention

Royal Society for the Prevention of Accidents (ROSPA)
Cannon House, The Priory Queensway, Birmingham B4 6BS
(Tel: 021–200–2461)
For information and teaching materials and regular journals on road, home, water, sports, leisure and work safety and safety in education.

Child Accident Prevention Trust (CAPT)
28 Portland Place, London W1N 4DE   (Tel: 071–636–2545)
For all aspects of child accidents and provision of research papers, fact sheets and pamphlets.

Parliamentary Advisory Council for Transport Safety (PACTS)
c/o Department of Civil Engineering, Imperial College, South Kensington, London SW7 2BU   (Tel: 071–589–5111 ext 4831)
For activities relating to the parliamentary process covering all aspects of transport accidents.

Medical Commission on Accident Prevention (MCAP)
c/o Royal College of Surgeons, 35–43 Lincoln's Inn Fields, London WC2A 3PN   (Tel: 071–242–3176)
For many aspects of accidents including roads, work and home, the effects of alcohol and drugs, falls in the elderly.

Department of Trade and Industry (DTI)
Consumer Safety Unit, 10–18 Victoria Street, London SW1H 0NN
(Tel: 071–215–7877)
For home and leisure accidents.

Department of Transport (DOT)
2 Marsham Street, London SW1P 3EB
For road traffic accidents.

Transnet*
16 Warren Lane, London SE18 6DW   (Tel: 081–854–5425)

Transport 2000*
Walkden House, 10 Melton Street, London NW1 2EJ

*Pressure groups working for improvements in the national transport system in relation to social, health, economic and environmental factors.

9 Occupational disease

The association between disease and occupation has been known since the earliest times. One of the earliest occupations, mining, was known to be hazardous not only because of accidents but also because of respiratory disease. Thus, in Roman and pre-medieval times only convicts and slaves were employed in such work—*proxima morti poena coercito*—a sentence to the mines was as good as the death penalty. However, little attention was paid to the health of workers until Bernardino Ramazzini, Professor of Medicine at Padua University, published *De Morbis Artificum* in 1700, and described a wide range of occupational diseases.[1] Later, the industrial revolution brought with it horrific conditions in factories and mines leading to high morbidity and mortality. During this period the major problems of occupational disease developed such as lead poisoning in the potteries and in paint manufacture, 'phossy jaw' in match making using white phosphorus, and pneumoconiosis in miners. Whilst many of these classical occupational diseases have now been virtually eliminated, the introduction of new technology and changing patterns of employment has led to new problems such as occupational deafness and occupational asthma.

The substantial loss of traditional heavy, dirty industrial jobs such as in shipyards, steel foundries and mines has been balanced by growth in the service, retail and leisure industries (Fig. 9.1). With robotics and automation, the machine operator or tradesman has substituted a visual display terminal for his tools. The increasing employment of women has brought with it new concerns, for example' the effects of work on reproductive performance. Although work is much safer and healthier than in the past, paradoxically there is growing public concern about hazards in the workplace.

Occupational disease and ill health in Britain today

As new occupational diseases are recognised, eg viral hepatitis in hospital staff, occupational asthma, occupational deafness, angiosarcoma of the liver, and vibration white finger, they have been added to the list of prescribed diseases, and have become eligible for benefit. In the UK, in 1988, 5,670 people were awarded benefit for having a 'prescribed disease', the majority being occupational lung disease and occupational deafness. The criteria for these awards in most cases are very stringent in terms of proof of exposure and the extent of disability and therefore

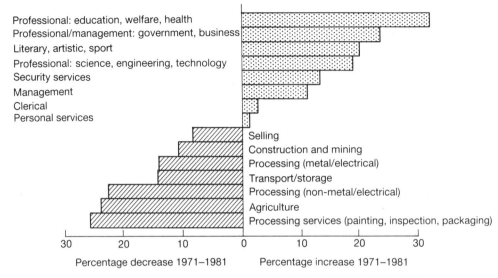

Fig. 9.1 *Change in employment by occupation. England and Wales, 1971–81.* Source: *OPCS.*

only measure severe disease. Within the lung disease category the traditional occupational dust diseases are declining (with the exception of mesothelioma), but the relatively recently included occupational asthma is not, with increasing recognition of causes of this disease.

Benefit changes in 1984 reduced claims for several other diseases, but there is probably a genuine decline in most, except vibration white finger.

Information sources

The early occupational diseases were specific to occupation and were clearly identified as being caused by exposure to harmful physical, chemical and biological hazards in the workplace. Thus the beat diseases, for example, prepatellar bursitis (widely known as housemaid's knee, but more common in miners), the acute poisonings, and infections such as anthrax, were recognised early. Mortality statistics and industrial injury awards indicate that most of these disorders are now declining, although some diseases with a long latency such as meso-thelioma, which may occur up to 40 years after the last substantial environmental exposure, still occur. Information on trends in occupational diseases is available from the annual reports of benefit awards under the Industrial Injuries Scheme administered by the Department of Social Security (Table 9.1).[2]

Limited information is also available from the reporting scheme under the Reporting of Diseases and Dangerous Occurrence Regulations (RIDDOR) whereby employers are supposed to report occurrences of certain occupational diseases. However, in the year 1988/89, only 296 cases of the limited list of diseases were reported. These included only 53 cases of vibration white finger although benefit was paid to 1,366 claimants for this condition.

Recognition of occupational disease is an important function of occupational health services. However, the provision and quality of such services is variable and about 40% of the workforce in the UK has no such service.[3] Recognition therefore is frequently dependent on the general practitioner or hospital physician who may have had little or no training or experience in occupational medicine, familiarity with occupational diseases, or of which diseases are notifiable. A voluntary scheme for the surveillance of work related and occupational respiratory disease (SWORD) has suggested the true frequency of disease may be three times greater than previously reported.[4]

It is likely that the official statistics on occupational disease in Britain seriously underestimate the real occurrence of these diseases.

Under-reporting of occupational disease can be attributed to:

- the stringent criteria for compensation under the Industrial Injuries Scheme;
- failure of reporting under RIDDOR;
- lack of awareness in the community and medical profession.

Taking into account under-reporting, it has been estimated that the incidence of occupational disease in the UK is approximately one case for every 4,000 employees.[5] Comparison with other countries reveals that the rate in Sweden is one case for 170 employees; one case for 500 in the USA; and one case for 7,400 in the Netherlands. However, these differences are probably due to the provision of occupational health services (highest in Sweden) and the varying criteria for diagnosis of occupational disease and its recording. The European Commission has recommended that a common schedule of occupational diseases be adopted throughout the Community as a basis for future information gathering and prevention.

Occupationally related ill-health

Largely unmeasured is the growing number of other diseases, not specific to occupation, but recognised as sometimes having an occupational component. Some of the common illnesses which may be

Table 9.1 New cases of occupational disease diagnosed under the Industrial Injuries and Pneumoconiosis, Byssinosis and Miscellaneous Diseases Benefit Schemes.[2]

A. Occupational lung diseases and deafness

	Disablement benefit — Year										
	1978	1979	1980	1981	1982	1983	1984	1985	1986	1987	1988
Pneumoconiosis (except asbestosis)	665	725	665	657	611	540	451	468	480	469	411
Asbestosis	132	135	150	153	185	212	200	301	329	282	225
Byssinosis	79	76	156	113	135	74	63	37	27	25	15
Farmer's lung	2	10	14	12	11	8	4	6	11	8	15
Occupational asthma (3)	x	x	x	x	105	175	136	170	171	202	222
Mesothelioma	..	..	..	93	123	148	201	245	305	399	479
Lung cancer (asbestos) (3)	x	x	x	x	x	x	x	8	34	55	59
Lung cancer (nickel)	1	1	2	–	–	1	5	2	3	–	–
Bilateral pleural thickening (3)	x	x	x	x	x	x	x	61	111	115	114
Other occupational lung disease	4	5	9	3	9	6	1	2	5	10	5
Occupational deafness (1)	527	555	331	1022	680	447	1443	1464	1179	1381	1515
Total	*1410*	*1507*	*1657*	*2053*	*1859*	*1611*	*2504*	*2764*	*2655*	*2946*	*3060*

B. Other diseases

| | Year | | | | | | | | | | |
| | Injury and disablement benefit (5) | | | | | | Disablement benefit (6) | | | | |
	1977/78	78/79	79/80	80/81	81/82	83/83 (4)	83/84	84/85	85/86	86/87 (2)	87/88 (2)
Dermatitis	7651	7004	5816	3960	3452	2110	611	619	785	464	368
Tenosynovitis	3537	3259	3009	2413	2282	1433	337	390	619	376	322
Vibration white finger (3)	x	x	x	x	x	x	x	3	641	1366	1673
Beat conditions	952	765	734	621	525	324	131	180	220	57	171
Viral hepatitis	31	25	32	40	26	24	3	5	9	5	3
Tuberculosis	72	44	39	32	29	11	6	7	3	13	3
Leptospirosis	4	2	3	7	1	4	2	–	–	1	–
Other infections	38	28	11	9	2	3	2	–	1	5	–
Poisonings	33	37	29	23	30	14	2	4	3	9	2
Occupational cancers	17	19	21	15	6	5	8	6	12	27	29
Other conditions	167	130	84	73	55	35	22	15	27	58	39
Total	*12,502*	*11,313*	*9778*	*7193*	*6408*	*3963*	*1124*	*1229*	*2320*	*2381*	*2610*

Source DSS

Symbols: – Series affected by change in prescription or benefit rules; . not available; x not applicable.

1. For occupational deafness, figures to 1982 are for years ending in June; for 1983 ending December: from 1984 years ending September.
2. From October 1986 disablement benefit was paid only for cases with disability assessed at 14% or more: the figures for 1986/87 and 1987/88 include cases not qualifying for benefit but assessed at 1–13%.
3. The following diseases were first prescribed during the period covered by the table

	Benefit first payable
Occupational asthma	1982
Lung cancer (asbestos)	1985
Bilateral pleural thickening	1985
Vibration white finger	1984/85

Table 9.2 Some common illnesses which may be occupational

Psychological	*Cardiovascular*
Stress	Ischaemic heart disease
Anxiety	Raynaud's phenomenon
Depression	
Phobias	*Neurological*
	Neuropathy
Musculoskeletal	Parkinsonism
Back pain	Dementia
Tenosynovitis	
Upper limb disorders	*Deafness*
Dermatological	*Cancer*
Dermatitis	Respiratory
Acne	Renal
Vitiligo	Liver
Hyperpigmentation	Leukaemia
	Bladder
	Skin
Respiratory	
Upper respiratory tract irritation	
Asthma	
Bronchitis	
Emphysema	

occupational in origin or in certain individuals are listed in Table 9.2. All human systems can be affected by work and indeed occupationally related ill-health may also be a great mimic of other conditions. The size of this problem is hard to judge because of difficulty in identifying the occupational link in individual cases.

Thus, the patient or employee with recurrent upper respiratory symptoms and headaches may be suffering from the effect of work in an inadequately ventilated or humidified office; asthma of recent origin may be due to a new workplace exposure; common skin problems such as dermatitis, acne, pigmentation changes, and infections can be occupational; much musculoskeletal morbidity, such as back pain, cervical spondylosis, and tenosynovitis is work related; recurrent dyspepsia may be related to shift work or vague abdominal discomfort due to lead poisoning; deafness in an elderly man may be due to 40 years working in a foundry rather than age; cancer in some sites may be work related. Psychological problems are common in the employed and stress-related disorders would seem to be increasing as all sections of industry, including the medical profession, are perpetually engaged in the quest for greater efficiency and productivity. Whilst occupational factors in anxiety depression and 'burn-out' are easily identifiable, other organically based but related problems such as the post-viral fatigue syndrome seem to be becoming more prevalent. Many of these common health problems are not identified as occupational even when a relationship to work can be identified.

Cancer

It has been estimated that occupation accounts for about 5,000 cancer deaths per year in England and Wales,[6] yet in 1987 industrial death benefit was paid in only 909 deaths, and of these the majority were for dust related lung disease and asbestos. Occupational cancers are also discussed in Chapter 6.

Back pain and musculoskeletal disorders

Back pain and other musculoskeletal syndromes are the commonest conditions with a significant occupational component, which is, however, generally hard to quantify or confirm. Low back pain will occur in about 80% of the population, mostly during some time in their working life. The epidemiology of back pain in industry has been defined and the high risk industries and occupations are well known, for example mining and labouring. The prevalence of back pain differs only marginally between heavy and light occupations but the degree of disability which occurs is twice as great in heavy occupations. Back problems have significant economic effect with lost production in 1982–83 estimated as in excess of £1,000 million.[7] The size of the problem and the fact that there is no instant treatment have led to much effort being expended in the pursuit of prevention of back pain within industry, by pre-employment screening, by training workers in manual handling and by the application of ergonomic principles to the task design.

Training is faithfully performed in most industries, but there is little evidence that one or two days training in lifting is of any greater benefit in improving the lifting technique of the worker than would be a two-day training programme to perfect a golf swing.

Some individual risk factors for back pain have been identified such as height, weight, strength and the size of the spinal canal, but pre-employment screening is not yet established as effective.[8]

The occupational risk factors can be more easily modified. These include avoiding lifting heavy loads in confined environments, avoiding the need to perform a bending twisting method, eliminating tripping and stumbling hazards, and avoiding frequent repetitions of heavy lifting. In these ways, hazards to the back can be designed out of many work environments.

A large number of other musculoskeletal problems can be caused by work using high force with frequent repetitive movements. The wrist and forearm are prone to tendon problems such as tenosynovitis, stenosing tenosynovitis, de Quervain's disease, especially if such work involves flexion, hyper-extension or deviation of the wrist with the fingers either clenched or spread widely. Entrapment neuropathy such as carpal tunnel syndrome is also common with repetitive manual work. Thus studies have suggested that 53% of Finnish butchers had carpal tunnel syndrome, 18% of Swedish scissor workers and 56% of Swedish packers had tendon lesions and in a poultry processing plant 12.8% of workers had problems over one year.

Repetitive strain injury is a generic term which has become popular in recent years. It tends to be used by the lay public to describe a number of upper limb disorders including the specific entities mentioned above and any cause of pain in the upper limb, shoulder or neck which is apparently associated with work activity. There is sometimes little proven pathology, the diagnosis may be uncertain, and it may be difficult to separate the physical and psycho-social causal factors. An example of the latter was the massive epidemic of repetitive strain injury which swept Australia in the early 1980s following the introduction of visual display units and electronic keyboards. In other societies where there has been a controlled rate of introduction of such new technology, the provision of appropriate training and good workplace design, and a satisfactory psycho-social work environment, problems occur much less frequently.

However, there can be no doubt that such disorders of the upper limb are common, cause much sickness absence, are probably increasing, and are largely preventable.

The skin

The skin is a very common site of occupational ill-health, the problems ranging from physical trauma, to dermatitis and carcinoma. Dermatitis is usually irritant, although some cases can be allergic with numerous causes such as nickel and chrome salts, epoxy resins, substances used in rubber maufacture, antibiotic manufacture, hairdressing dyes, and plant products especially the primula group. Pitch and tar may cause darkening of the skin as will arsenic and mercury poisoning. On the other hand vitiligo and depigmentation occur with some exposure to phenols. The cancer risks of excessive exposure to sunlight are an occupational risk to some groups such as farmers and fishermen.

Liver and kidney

The liver and kidney share a vulnerability to many toxic agents. Liver failure can be precipitated by the chlorinated hydrocarbons such as carbon tetrachloride and chloroform. The kidney is especially susceptible to heavy metals including lead, mercury, cadmium, gold, thallium and uranium.

Central nervous system

Neurotoxic effects, ie damage to motor or sensory nerves or other parts of the nervous system, can occur with workplace exposure to heavy metals such as lead, mercury, thallium and arsenic, organic solvents and numerous other chemicals. Mercury poisoning used to be common in the hat industry leading to the aphorism 'mad as a hatter'. Although eliminated in that industry, mercury poisoning can occur in the laboratory technicians or dentists who have exposure to mercury amalgam.

Exposure to solvents may produce a mild intoxicating effect and there is increasing evidence that toluene sniffing may produce permanent brain damage and dementia. The evidence that brain damage occurs as a result of occupational exposure to solvents is relatively weak.

Cardiovascular disease

A number of occupational exposures have been shown to increase the risk of cardiovascular disease. Most jobs now have reduced physical activity as a result of mechanisation, automation and changing work practices. However, work with chemicals such as carbon-disulphide, used in the viscose rayon manufacture, rubber and chemical industries is associated with increase in coronary heart disease. Other solvents such as trichloroethylene or 1,1,1-trichloroethane can precipitate cardiac arrhythmias and sudden death. Methylene chloride, a common ingredient in paint strippers, which causes the formation of carboxy-haemoglobin in the body (similar to carbon-monoxide poisoning) has also been reported to cause sudden death. Dynamite manufacturing involves exposure of the workers to nitro-glycerine and it has also been associated with the risk of angina and sudden death when the worker is away from work. Nitro-glycerine is of course related to the nitrate drugs used for angina and its likely effect on the heart is that of reflex vasoconstriction of the coronary arteries after withdrawal from exposure to nitro-glycerine and its vasodilatory effects. Hypertension has been associated with occupational exposure to noise and vibration.

The population at risk of particular occupation-related illnesses may be quite large. For example, Raynaud's phenomenon, the cold induced white finger due to underlying vascular damage, is common and associated with many medical conditions, but is also a presenting sign of vibration induced injury—vibration white finger. A large survey by the Health and Safety Executive showed that about 426,000 workers in manufacturing and construction industries, public utilities, agriculture and forestry use tools which expose them to hand/arm vibration, and of these 152,000 used such tools for relatively long periods.[5]

Principles of prevention

Identifying the hazard

Identifying the hazard is relatively easy when there is a specific and well understood relationship between the work exposure and the disease, but much more difficult when the association is weak. The vast majority of occupational disease has first been identified through astute clinical observations. For example, Percival Pott was the first to identify an occupational cancer when he described scrotal cancer in chimney sweeps in 1775. Discovery of the link between wood dust and nasal cancer occurred when Esme Hadfield, an observant otolaryngologist recognised that a number of uncommon nasal tumours had occurred in men all employed in the furniture making industry.[9]

While routine surveillance of mortality and morbidity records rarely leads to the identification of a new occupational hazard, there is a wide variety of morbidity and mortality data collected by employers, government departments, hospitals and workplaces which may be useful in detecting unusual patterns of ill-health or deaths. For example, the national mortality data reveal significant differences in death rates between occupational groups much of which are probably due to social factors, but occupation is also relevant. A survey of workers working with dyestuff intermediates revealed a large number of cases of bladder cancer and suggested that benzidine and naphthylamines were the likeliest causes.[10]

Once a link is suspected, further epidemiology is needed to establish its nature and extent. This may not be easy especially for less objectively measured diseases. While under-recognition of occupational illness is certainly common, individuals or groups will often attempt to prove that any ill-health is due to a new work environment or that a new work location is harmful. This in itself can cause much confusion, encourage mass psychogenic illness and complicate the identification of the real health problems which may arise with changing work practices.

Thus, carefully designed and executed epidemiological studies are often necessary to identify whether or not there is a causal relationship between working environment and ill-health.

Screening of chemicals and toxicology

Identification of the hazard through observation of the disease is only possible after people become ill, and primary prevention — by identification of the potential hazard — is clearly preferable. Animal and laboratory testing of many chemicals for potential harmful effects such as mutagenicity, cytogenicity and carcinogenicity is undertaken but the significance to humans of such testing is not always clear. These procedures may prevent problems, but we only find out about failures of the system.

Risk assessment

Even when a hazard has been established it must still be recognised in a particular workplace and the risk assessed. Failure to do so can cause significant problems for example, when engineers at sea cleaned out the oil fired boilers and became ill because no-one had recognised that the boiler-soot scale contained vanadium pentoxide, or when building maintenance men disturbed insulation material and created dust, without using protective equipment or establishing that the material was asbestos. Thus, every workplace requires assessment of the risk of substances and processes before work commences and this is now a duty under the Control of Substances Hazardous to Health Regulations, 1988 (see below).

The risk posed by a hazardous substance depends on its route into the body and the extent of exposure. Evaluation of such hazards require:

- detailed understanding of the substances used;
- how substances will be handled;
- what processes are employed, and
- measurement where necessary of the levels of dust, fumes, gases, liquids, mists and sprays and comparison with recommended standards.

Such measurements and assessment of risk are often undertaken by specialists in occupational hygiene, who have the skills and measuring techniques to quantify and evaluate risk.

These assessments of risk to workers, sometimes called 'Environmental Impact Assessments', are being incorporated into more holistic appraisals of an industrial activity. This approach, used in progressive industries, can be applied to new buildings, plants, industrial processes and products. Before any new manufacturing processes are made operational or a product introduced for the market place, a full assessment is made of all the materials used, the risks, hazards, waste produced by the process, how there might be a risk to the worker, or to the user of the end product. This assessment can be extended to cover product disposal, eg how can it be disposed of safely without hazard to individuals or to the environment? In some industries this procedure is laid down as a routine and is done not only for the prevention of occupational disease but also to understand the implications of the process for the general environment, ie from cradle to grave. Such assessments if done thoroughly and with vigour can do much to aid the primary prevention of occupational disease and can systematically identify all risks and necessary control procedures.

Control of the hazard

Ideally, the hazard should be eliminated from the workplace but this is not always possible. Figure 9.2 shows the traditional hierarchy of control: elimination, substitution, enclosure, segregation, personal protective equipment.

Environmental concerns may conflict with these principles. For example, chlorofluorocarbons (CFCs) were substituted for methyl bromide refrigerants and for other solvents used for cleaning components in the electronic and other industries precisely because they are relatively non-toxic, non-flammable and safe. Some environmentally friendly

> • Eliminate the hazardous material
>
> • Substitute the hazardous material
>
> • Enclose the process (eg exhaust ventilation)
>
> • Segregate the workplace
>
> • Provide personal protective equipment

Fig. 9.2 *Heirarchy of control of occupational hazard.*

chemicals are not very people friendly and so care has to be taken to balance the requirement for individual health and safety with that of a sustainable environment.

Monitoring effectiveness of control

Exposure limits in the work place

Currently, in the UK there are two categories of limits published by the Health and Safety Executive:

i   *Maximum Exposure Levels*: these give the maximum concentration for inhalation over a specified response period.
ii *Occupational Exposure Standards*: these define the concentration average for the reference period, and if they are exceeded a strategy of reduction must be identified.

There are also limits for substances which can be absorbed through the skin. However, these limits are derived from the pool of available knowledge, some on the basis of studies undertaken many years ago. As new information emerges limits may be changed; for example, the recent reduction of dose limits for radiation workers and of the acceptable levels for asbestos in the air.

Epidemiological studies are often necessary to establish dose–response relationships and thus the appropriate exposure standard. A classical example of such work in recent years is that carried out by the Institute of Occupational Medicine in Edinburgh in the field of pneumoconiosis, where the dose–response relationship between coal workers' pneumoconiosis and coal dust levels was established and which led to the

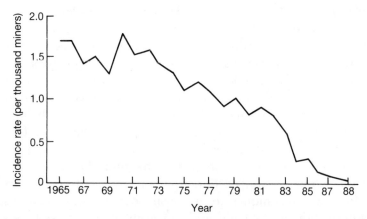

Fig. 9.3 *The incidence rate of pneumoconiosis certifications per thousand miners between 1965 and 1988. The incidence rate for 1988 was 0.08 per thousand.* Source: *Ref. 12.*

introduction of new and lower dust standards in coal mines throughout the world.[11] As a result, there has been a striking fall in incidence rates of certification of pneumoconiosis in working miners[12] (Fig. 9.3).

The control limits are set for the majority but in any population there may be individuals who are particularly susceptible to an occupational hazard. This may be due to working practices, eg a poor lifting technique, which increase the risk of back pain; to personal habits, eg nail biting which leads to ingestion of lead; or to individual biological susceptibility, eg atopy predisposing to the development of allergic eczema.

Monitoring

Having established controls, it is important to check that they work. Epidemiological studies, such as the analysis of mortality differences in occupations or in geographical areas, and the published statistics on occupational injuries and ill-health, are all useful long-term measures of control of disease, but the analysis of health surveillance results in working populations may be more immediately useful. Unfortunately, even with reasonable adherence to occupational exposure limits and control procedures, occupational diseases may still not be adequately controlled. One example is occupational deafness which is regarded as one of the ten leading occupational diseases in the US, yet a recent review suggests that prevention is currently inadequate.[13]

While reduction of noise levels in industry to 80 decibels would virtually eliminate occupational risk, present preventive strategies are to reduce noise levels to 85 decibels and if this is not achieved to protect the exposed worker with ear muffs or ear plugs and to monitor the success or otherwise of the protective programme by regular measurement of hearing levels by audiometry. However, hearing levels deteriorate with age and audiometry is a very imprecise tool. Diagnosis of noise-induced hearing loss continues to rise as do claims for compensation. Thus, the traditional use of secondary prevention techniques (regular measurement of hearing levels in the workforce) is only partially effective and ultimately the most efficient way to prevent occupational deafness is to employ primary prevention, ie to eliminate the hazard.

In such circumstances, the role of the occupational health professional remains clear—to create and maintain a database of noise exposures and hearing levels, to encourage and monitor the use of hearing protection, to monitor and encourage engineering control, and through epidemiological techniques to establish dose-response relationships and advise industry, society and government about what are the desirable working conditions.

Early detection of occupational disease

With many occupational diseases early recognition can reverse or diminish the disease process and thus early detection is vital. Screening can be established for occupational disease or for occupational related illness, to measure biological exposure or any biological effect. Epidemiological methods also help in early detection by effective surveillance of a working population and by selective examinations of workers at risk.

Pre-employment screening

Where there are particular hazards, or physical demands, pre-employment health assessment may be necessary. For most occupations a pre-employment questionnaire is perfectly adequate. The purpose of a medical assessment of fitness for work is to make sure that an individual is fit to perform the task without risk to his own or others' health and safety. Its main aim is to ensure satisfactory job placement rather than exclude individuals who have a disability. It is the common experience that workers who have a disability are usually highly motivated and have excellent work and attendance records. Health advice may be needed when an individual's condition may limit or prevent him performing the job effectively (eg musculoskeletal condition that limits ability, manual handling or ability to lift heavy objects); when a condition might be made worse by the job (eg exposure to certain allergens in an asthmatic or excessive physical work in an individual with a cardiac problem); when a condition may make it unsafe to do a job (eg liability to unconsciousness in a hazardous situation, significant risk of deafness in someone who is already hearing impaired); when a condition is likely to make it unsafe for both the individual and others (eg vehicle driving of someone liable to sudden unconsciousness); or when a condition might be a hazard for the community (eg active gastrointestinal infection in a food handler).

A further important role of pre-employment health examination may be to establish a baseline for future comparison; for example audiometry before employment in a job with high noise exposure; chest X-ray in a prospective mine worker; hepatitis B antigen in those working in a renal dialysis unit.

The medical standards which apply to any particular occupation may be either advisory or may have a statutory basis. Examples of the latter are the examinations required by law for those being considered for work as divers, pilots, coal miners and in the fire service.

Biological monitoring

The scope, frequency and nature of health surveillance of a working population must be based on the nature and extent of risks. Examinations should focus on the target organs of a specific hazard, eg chest X-ray in coal miners; audiometry in a noise-exposed worker; blood, lead and urine coproporphyrin in a lead worker; measurement of trichloracetic acid in the urine of those exposed to trichlorethylene; measurement of lung function (FEVI and FVC) in a worker exposed to isocyanates. Health surveillance may therefore range from a questionnaire, a blood, urine or lung function test, a limited examination by a nurse or a full physical examination.

Monitoring has become highly sophisticated; as knowledge of the metabolism of chemicals in the body has advanced, tests have developed which can measure whether the exposure is recent or not, and the amounts stored in an organ, in the whole body, or bound to the target molecule. While measurements of a chemical in the urine, blood or expired air are most commonly performed, analysis of hair, nails, fat and teeth can be used in some circumstances.

Less specific tests such as the assessment of mutagenic activity in the urine of rubber workers or nurses handling cytotoxic drugs are of less value in individuals but may be used to assess groups at risk if compared to other groups of unexposed controls.

Increasingly, tests are being developed which can demonstrate the effect at very low levels of exposure to chemicals, and examples of these are immuno-toxicological assays.

Genetic toxicology which involves measuring change in DNA molecules, is becoming more readily available for workers exposed to industrial carcinogens and mutagens. Recently, measurement of oncogene proteins in the serum has been used to identify workers at risk of developing cancer. Although these tests are still experimental and not yet conclusive, considerable advances in these screening techniques may be anticipated and with them the ability to identify very early those individuals who may be at special risk. If so, there may be the opportunity of prevention, by removing them from exposure.

Such biological surveillance should always take second place to the identification, evaluation and control of the hazard, and monitoring workplace health is only justified if there is not complete confidence in the adequate control of the hazard.

Legal framework

The evolution of health and safety legislation since the Health and Morals of Apprentices Act (1802) has underpinned much of the substantial progress in the reduction of occupational disease.

The Health and Safety at Work Act in 1974 replaced much piecemeal legislation and established the Employment Medical Advisory Service whose duty is to give advice to anyone in all matters concerning the effect of work on health, and health on work. Under the terms of the Health and Safety at Work Act, specific responsibilities relating to health and safety are placed upon both employer and employee. More recently, further regulations under the Act (the Control of Substances Hazardous to Health (COSHH) Regulations 1988) have reinforced the principle of assessment of risk and installation of control measures before any potential hazardous material can be used. Control measures also have to be monitored and these may include health surveillance. Thus the legislation in this field assists the primary and secondary prevention of occupational disease. Specific regulations also cover diving, radioactive substances, carcinogenic substances and other hazardous substances or occupations.

A further important legal duty is the common law duty of the employer who must take such care of his employees as is 'reasonably practicable'. 'Practicable' means that some action is physically possible and 'reasonably practicable' that the nature and extent of this risk to health must be weighed against the cost and effectiveness of measures taken to eliminate it. The injured employee or bereaved family has thus the option, under common law, of suing the employer if it is believed that the employer was negligent.

However, in addition to the legal constraint many employers rightly see good health and safety as good business, and organisations which take a robust approach to the quality control of their products, and processes, usually also view health and safety as quality issues.

Health promotion in industry

Health eduction and promotion is one of the roles of occupational health services and in recent years many companies have developed extensive programmes, some of which are far more comprehensive than those available in the general community. The workplace provides excellent opportunities for a wide range of preventive activities which are not directly concerned with work related disease and injury. These programmes usually involve the tripartite approach of education screening and action plans to enable individuals to participate in specific programmes to deal with risks which have been identified or lifestyle issues which they may wish to address. The programmes that have been established can include:

- the provision of smoke-free work places
- smoking cessation clinics

- alcohol and drug treatment policies
- publicised healthy eating campaigns in work-place cafeterias
- health checks
- provision of fitness training facilities and exercise classes
- lifestyle management courses
- stress counselling.

Many companies have chosen to invest actively in this area without waiting for proof from the scientific community that such pro-active measures are necessarily worthwhile. They are provided and perceived as an employee benefit and an aid to employee well-being and morale. In the UK some of the most intensive and complete examples of health promotion can be seen in companies as varied as Marks and Spencer, the Post Office and IBM UK. Marks and Spencer for example has performed screening for cervical cancer since 1968 and mammography since 1973 with at least 80% of all female employees participating. The Post Office has developed a high profile Health Promotion programme including screening with, for example, a Health Bus to visit their many locations. IBM UK offers all employees a periodic health risk appraisal and multiphasic screen, linked to health education. It has found that the majority of its employees are aware of their personal risk factors such as cholesterol and blood pressure, and that, following the implementation of screening, their health care costs for ill health were lower than expected in 1989. Whilst such programmes have received little critical evaluation in the UK, evidence of their benefit has been accepted elsewhere.[14]

CONCLUSIONS AND RECOMMENDATIONS

The prevention of occupational disease is one of the success stories of prevention in Britain but the challenge of the less definitely occupationally related diseases remains, as do the dramatic differences in death rates between the various occupational groups. While these differences may be due more to the social characteristics of the individuals employed, unravelling the various components of any such differences is a major challenge.

To further the prevention of occupational disease and ill health there is a need for:

1   More information by improved occupational mortality data, and by developing a new and more comprehensive system of reporting

of industrial disease, by employers and medical practitioners. The present systems are inadequate.

2   More *ad hoc* surveys and 'spotter' general practices.

3   Improved evaluation of possible control measures, especially in such major causes of morbidity as the musculoskeletal disorders and back pain.

4   Finally, there is an urgent need to improve the awareness and knowledge of the medical profession. Basic medical training does not include much occupational medicine. Medical practitioners, at least must be trained to ask the following questions of themselves or the patient who presents with a condition which might be related to occupation:

- What is your occupation and job history?
- How did this happen?
- Could it have been prevented?

10 Childhood

Introduction

This chapter aims to demonstrate the role prevention has played in the dramatic improvements in child health over the last few decades and outlines prospects for the future. It also highlights the fundamental role that social factors play in health and disease and the difficulty of considering child health in isolation, separated from the social or family context. Many childhood health problems are preventable, more often through changes in society and the environment, and in social (and political) attitudes to children and social disadvantage, than through 'health service' actions.

Some current preventive activities in childhood, such as immunisations, are of proven benefit. Others, including much developmental screening, are of uncertain benefit. Critical evaluation of current programmes is a priority need, especially in view of the recent move to encourage general practitioners to take the major role in preventive health care, including child surveillance, and the expectation that services provided will be cost-effective.

In this section topics covered elsewhere in this report, eg immunisation against infectious diseases (Chapter 7) or accident prevention (Chapter 8), will not be considered in depth, nor will prenatal diagnosis and genetic screening, which has been the subject of a recent Royal College of Physicians report.[1]

By many criteria, child health in the United Kingdom has improved enormously over the last 70–80 years. Many infectious diseases and other conditions have been controlled or prevented, and there has been a dramatic and continuing reduction in the likelihood that a baby will die around the time of birth, during the first year or in later childhood (Fig. 10.1).

Certain previously damaging or life-threatening conditions, such as rheumatic fever, have largely disappeared from affluent countries like the UK. Nevertheless, many illnesses causing death or disability remain and certain disorders appear to be increasing in incidence, for example, diabetes, asthma and eczema, possibly associated with changes in the environment. Advances in medical care have resulted in an increased prevalence of serious chronic conditions as more children survive with previously fatal conditions. Even where such children are subsequently well or cured (eg from cancer, renal failure or serious congenital heart conditions), the period of active treatment often puts

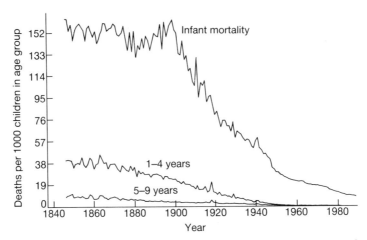

Fig. 10.1 *Mortality in infants and children, England and Wales 1846–1989.* Source: *OPCS.*

great stress on the families and on health care providers. These changes in the pattern of serious chronic disorders emphasise the need for primary prevention through the identification of causal processes in the initiation of the conditions, as well as for secondary prevention to identify problems as early as possible to ensure disability is minimised, and for tertiary prevention to minimise handicap during and subsequent to treatment.

As well as focussing on the reduction in serious acute paediatric problems and the rise in chronic paediatric problems, attention is being drawn increasingly to the prevention of less obvious health problems, including behaviour disorders, which may affect a child's opportunity to gain maximum benefit from education and to fulfil his or her potential as an individual, within a family and in the wider society.

Social and environmental disadvantage

A major area of opportunity for prevention, perhaps more through social change and political commitment than medical input, is the continuing health gap between advantaged and disadvantaged sections of the British population. This is particularly applicable to children. Compared with a child born into an advantaged family, a baby born into socially disadvantaged circumstances is much more at risk of a variety of health problems and of dying during early life. Although overall infant mortality rates (deaths in the first year) have reduced considerably, the differential in death rates between higher and lower social classes has remained virtually unchanged since 1950 (Fig. 10.2);

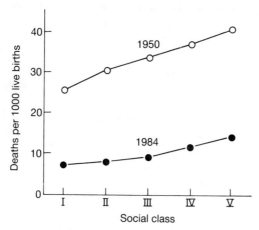

Fig. 10.2 *Infant mortality rates in 1980 and 1984 by father's social class.* Source: *OPCS.*

the increased rate in social class 5 families over social class 1 was 59% in 1950 and 77% in 1984. In most other similarly wealthy countries, these social differentials have been reduced or have disappeared.

The health problems associated with social and environmental disadvantage include respiratory illness, infections, accidents, behaviour problems and developmental delay, and such children are more likely to be hospitalised. Markers of disadvantage include extremes of maternal age, poor parental education, high birth order and unsupported mothers. Such adverse circumstances are often associated with emotional and financial difficulties. It is unlikely that these factors, of themselves, cause ill-health in children but they are linked with likely 'causal' factors such as nutritional problems, 'stress', and increased opportunities for cross infection associated with overcrowding and poor hygiene.

Social, environmental and biological factors may operate independently to cause ill-health but very often are interrelated. For example, very young mothers are more likely to have low educational attainment, to be unmarried and unsupported, to smoke, to be living in unsatisfactory housing and to experience other stressful life events. Thus, their children may be multiply disadvantaged. There is extensive information on this topic and recent reviews, often with strong recommendations for change.[2,3] There has however been little official action following these reports, particularly at a governmental level.

Improving social conditions and ensuring support for mothers and families are likely to be the most effective ways of preventing ill-health in childhood. Extended family or other social support and learning how to 'cope' may prevent some ill-effects of being disadvantaged.

Table 10.1 The effectiveness of some medical preventive activities in childhood

	Effective (benefit demonstrated)	**'Best bet'** (likely benefit but unconfirmed)
Prenatal	Rubella immunisation after screening Periconceptual vitamins (recurrent neural tube defects)	Review of maternal health/ obstetric record
Pregnancy	Screening for syphilis, hepatitis B Ultrasound scan for neural tube defects	Stopping maternal smoking Antenatal clinic attendance Avoid maternal drugs/ alcohol Chorionic villus sampling for thalassaemia, and some other inborn errors of metabolism
Newborn	Guthrie test for hypothyroidism and PKU Anti D, rhesus protection	Health promotion Haemoglobinopathy screening Congenital dislocation of the hip examination General physical examination Neonatal hearing test
Infancy	Avoidance of unmodified cow's milk Vitamin supplements Immunisations	Breast feeding Hearing check
Preschool	Immunisation booster	Development surveillance Responding to parental concern re vision, hearing and behavioural problems 'Healthy' diet

Table 10.1   *(continued)*

	Effective (benefit demonstrated)	**'Best bet'** (likely benefit but unconfirmed)

School	Vision screening	Health surveillance
		  including growth
		Identification of learning
		  disabilities
		Health promotion/
		  education
		Regular exercise

Adolescence	Immunisation booster	Health promotion/ education Regular exercise Birth control advice Safer sex

'Effective' and 'best bet' prevention

Prevention in the early years of life includes those preventions where benefit has been demonstrated and those where it remains unproven (Table 10.1). In the remainder of this chapter prevention will be considered in relation to avoidable death and selected causes of morbidity. Child health surveillance will be considered separately. The framework used to discuss preventive child health care is that summarised by John Butler in his excellent review of Child Health Surveillance in Primary Care,[4] shown in Fig. 10.3.

Perinatal and neonatal mortality: preventive aspects

Deaths in early life are most likely during the first year (Fig. 10.4), especially in the neonatal period (the first month of life). The improvement in infant mortality (deaths in the first year) in England and Wales over recent years is almost entirely attributable to a reduction in neonatal mortality, which in large part reflects improved technical care of pregnant and parturient women and newborn babies.

Figure 10.4 shows the marked decline over recent decades in perinatal mortality (still-births and deaths in the first week). This has been due largely to changes in social and demographic factors such as maternal age, family size and social class. For example, about one-quarter of the

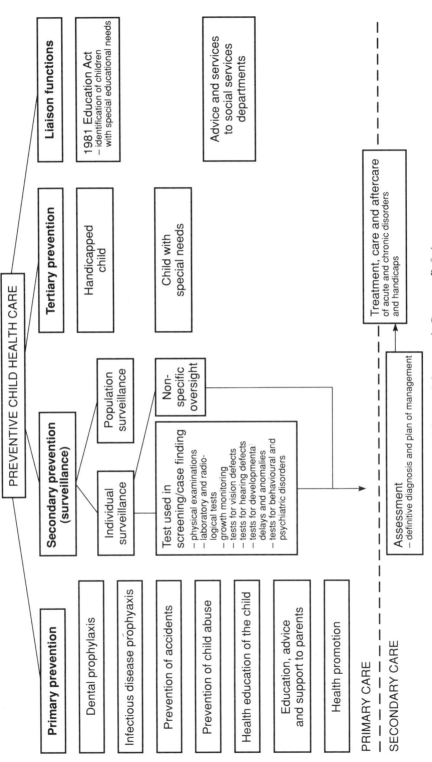

Fig. 10.3 *The preventive health care of preschool children: a definitional framework. Source: Ref. 4.*

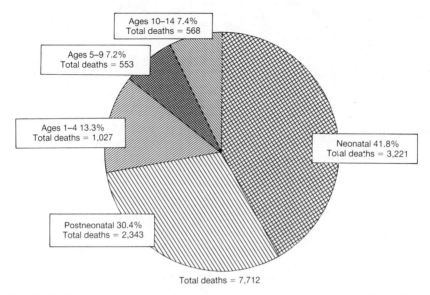

Fig. 10.4 *Distribution of deaths in childhood by age group, England and Wales 1990.*
Source: *OPCS.*

reduction in perinatal mortality rate between 1950 and 1973 in England
and Wales was associated with shifts in maternal age, parity and social
class.[5]

Family planning thus has an important role in the prevention of early
deaths and other health problems since mortality increases with
high parity, extremes of maternal age and short pregnancy intervals.
Termination of unwanted pregnancies in 'high risk' mothers is likely to
have contributed to the decline in perinatal mortality.

For some women, early detection of serious congenital or genetic
abnormalities by routine or targeted screening tests and/or ultrasound scanning provides the possibility of early termination of affected
pregnancies.

Maternal health and antenatal care. A healthy woman is likely to have a
healthy child. Women with medical conditions such as poorly controlled
diabetes or hypertension are at greater risk of pregnancy complications
and their babies have an increased risk of being born preterm and of
having problems in the newborn period. Good medical records, including
details of previous pregnancies, should identify obstetric risk factors
and provide the opportunity to initiate appropriate intervention. Thus
improved antenatal care will have some impact on perinatal mortality
in women with specific health problems requiring active management.

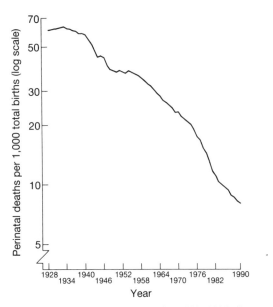

Fig. 10.5 *Perinatal mortality, England and Wales 1928–1990.* Source: *OPCS.*

However, for most women, the apparent benefit of early and more frequent antenatal care may largely reflect the type of mother who attends.

Birthweight. Overall, improvements in maternal health and social conditions have resulted in an increased average birthweight. However, the proportion of low birthweight babies (born <2500g) has remained virtually unchanged. Birthweight is the single most important predictor of perinatal mortality. For the years 1982–85 in England and Wales, 63% of still-births and deaths in the first week of life were born weighing less than 2500g. Low birthweight, associated with preterm delivery or with small size for gestational age (when there is often placental insufficiency), is also strongly associated with socio-economic deprivation. *Maternal smoking* is a major preventable factor in this relationship, with estimates showing a reduction of 10 grams in birth weight for each cigarette smoked per day during pregnancy (ie 200g lighter than predicted if a woman smokes an average of 20 cigarettes per day). The evidence linking low birthweight with subsequent developmental and educational problems makes avoidance of smoking in young women an important preventive health priority.

Preterm delivery is at least theoretically preventable and also contributes to infant morbidity and mortality. Associated factors include preeclamptic toxaemia which is also related to maternal cigarette smoking. Uncontrolled maternal hypertension increases the likelihood of placental abruption and poor fetal growth.

Delivery

Modern obstetric management has had an important beneficial impact on perinatal mortality and morbidity. This has been clearly documented in the 1970 compared with the 1958 National British Birth Cohort Study.[6,7] Maternal deaths and neurological damage in babies resulting from obstetric mishap are now rare and there is little evidence for the widespread belief that intrapartum care influences the likelihood of cerebral palsy. Cerebral palsy is not, in general, caused by birth asphyxia.[8] The prevention of most neurological damage in babies is likely to follow increased understanding of factors causing anatomical or physiological abnormalities which may manifest themselves in fetal or perinatal distress.

Caesarian section rather than vaginal delivery may be beneficial where labour is inevitable at less than 32 weeks gestation. Many obstetricians prefer caesarian section for breech deliveries at any gestational age although the evidence that this prevents brain damage remains equivocal. Overall, caesarian section delivery rates in the UK have increased over the last decade as they have in other countries,[9] often in the belief that brain damage is being prevented. Rates of 15% are not uncommon and in private practice can reach 30% or more. There may be disadvantages to mother and child from such operative intervention.

The importance of minimising administration of *drugs during labour* has been rightly stressed; up to 20 and on average 10 different medications have been recorded in North America. Short- and intermediate-term physiological and behavioural problems have been demonstrated in babies whose mothers were given analgesics, including epidural anaesthesia, during labour.[10]

The newborn

Developments in special care of the newborn and neonatal intensive care, with the availability of respiratory support, effective treatment of jaundice and infections and parenteral nutrition, have transformed the outcome for sick and especially very small infants and have prevented much mortality and morbidity. Even a technique as straightforward as naso-gastric tube feeding has prevented deaths and brain damage from starvation or the ill effects of low blood sugar. The pattern of

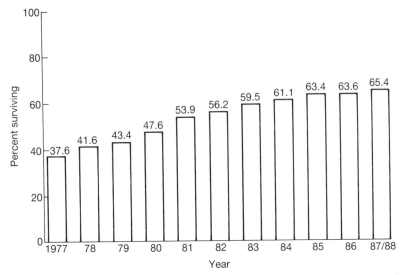

Fig. 10.6 *Percentage of very low weight (1500 g or less) births that survive more than one month.* Source: *OPCS.*

cerebral palsy has changed[11] in association with improved intact survival of moderately preterm babies (>28 weeks gestation) and the increasing survival of very preterm babies, some as immature as 23 weeks. This has implications for the prevalence of cerebral palsy in the childhood population.

Developments in the mechanical care of the newborn appear to be reaching their limits as reflected in the levelling off in survival rates of very low birthweight infants (Fig. 10.6).

More attention is now being placed on emotional and psychological factors. Optimal support and ideal environment are desirable for all mothers, but particularly for those who are most vulnerable so that bonding between the mother and child can be optimally effective.[12] The antenatal and newborn periods appear to be key times for health promotion which can include nutritional advice for mother and child, the need for social support and other preventive care.

Prevention and infant mortality

Although advances in medical care have contributed to the reduction in infant mortality seen this century (Fig. 10.1), the major impact has resulted from improvements in social and environmental conditions: better general nutrition, better water supplies and sewers, reduction in specific infections through immunisation and better access to fertility control. Unlike neonatal mortality, post-neonatal mortality (which has

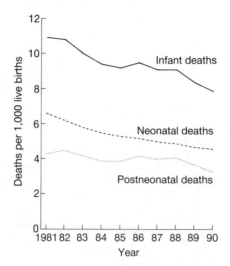

Fig. 10.7 *Infant mortality in England 1981–1990.* Source: *OPCS*.

a marked social class gradient) has shown little recent reduction (Fig. 10.7). This could be regarded as an indictment of social policy in regard to children and families.

Secular changes in the major causes of post-neonatal death (1 month to 1 year) from 1963 to 1987 are shown in Fig. 10.8. The most common cause is now sudden unexpected infant death, followed by congenital abnormalities and respiratory problems. The changing pattern in sudden infant death syndrome (SIDS) may in part reflect changing diagnostic criteria rather than an increase in this disorder, since there has been an associated fall in deaths attributed to respiratory conditions.

Sudden infant death syndrome is the commonest 'diagnosis' made when a baby dies between the ages of one month and one year. The cause of this condition remains unknown but is likely to be multifactorial. A specific diagnosis as to the cause of death can be made in some children labelled as 'cot deaths' when a careful post mortem is carried out by an experienced paediatric pathologist. There are preventive implications from some recent insights into possible causal mechanisms which include avoidance of overwrapping, parental smoking, prone lying position and infanticide. Attempts to identify babies at risk using check lists, with a view to preventing deaths by increased nursing and social support, have not proved widely successful. Many families use apnoea mattresses or other respiratory monitors for subsequent babies after one sibling has died, or use them following 'missed' cot deaths but there is no evidence of preventive benefit.[13]

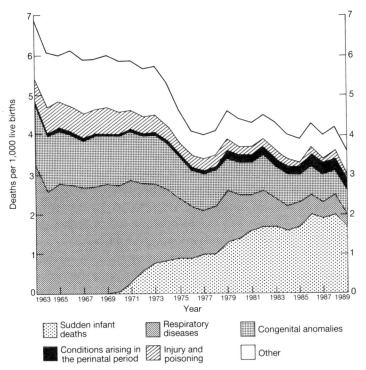

Fig. 10.8 *Cumulative postneonatal deaths by selected causes, England and Wales 1963–1989.* Source: *OPCS*.

Congenital abnormalities are an important cause of mortality and morbidity in early life and their significance has increased as control has been gained over infectious diseases. As many as 5% of live births show some genetic or developmental anomaly of varying severity and major malformations resulting in death or chronic handicap are present in about 2% of babies. Some known causes of congenital abnormality include chromosomal abnormalities, genetically inherited disorders and environmental factors such as ionising radiation or exposure to drugs, including alcohol, or infections in pregnancy, but in the majority of cases no clear-cut cause can be identified.

The scope for prevention of congenital abnormalities is therefore limited, but unnecessary radiographs should be avoided especially in pregnancy. Screening during pregnancy by ultrasound, amniocentesis and fetal or maternal blood samples is increasing and leading to the detection of some disorders with the possibility of termination of an affected pregnancy or early treatment.

Neural tube defects and other malformations, for example, cardiovascular or renal, can be identified by ultrasound. There has been a lessening of the early enthusiasm for intrauterine surgery undertaken to prevent damage, particularly of the renal tract, as it now is realised that many apparent abnormalities detected antenatally may resolve or improve after birth.[14] Further study is required.

Inherited disorders. Prenatal diagnosis and genetic screening, which is receiving increasing attention, has been the subject of a recent major College review and will not be considered in detail here. New developments will make the antenatal diagnosis of disorders such as cystic fibrosis and Duchenne muscular dystrophy possible so that the termination of an affected pregnancy becomes an option.

Haemoglobinopathies, eg thalassaemia, can be detected with chorionic villus sampling. This may be appropriate when parents have been identified as carriers. In southern Europe comprehensive thalassaemia control programmes have led to near eradication of new cases of this common and severe inherited disease.

Rhesus incompatibility is now a rare problem with anti-D immunoglobulin given immediately postnatally to rhesus negative mothers. However, an unacceptable number of cases are still being reported.

Congenital infections. Screening during pregnancy is important to detect *syphilis* and *hepatitis B* carriers so that treatment can be initiated. When a mother is identified as a hepatitis B carrier, early administration of immunoglobulin to the baby within hours of delivery followed by hepatitis B vaccine can prevent infection of the infant and the risk of persistent carriage of the virus with serious sequelae such as chronic hepatitis or hepatoma in later life. The benefit of routine screening for *toxoplasmosis* remains questionable in the UK where the prevalence of recognised congenital infection remains extremely low.[15] Screening for *cytomegalovirus* in pregnancy is not useful in the prevention of congenital abnormalities. Termination of a pregnancy complicated by infection would be the only option which would result in the loss of many normal fetuses and prevent the birth of only a small number of affected infants.[16]

Human immunodeficiency virus infection is an increasing problem. Universal voluntary antenatal screening is not recommended except in high prevalence areas, although selective testing is, for high risk groups. About one in five infants born to HIV positive mothers are themselves infected with the virus. Maternal HIV seropositivity is considered adequate grounds to terminate a pregnancy in terms of the 1967

Abortion Act. Related issues include consent to testing and the need for counselling services.[17]

Although routine *rubella* serological screening during pregnancy does not benefit the existing pregnancy it is important to identify women susceptible to infection so that they can be offered rubella vaccine in the postpartum period to protect subsequent pregnancies. However, any rash or contact with rubella during pregnancy must be fully investigated whether or not the woman has been vaccinated. Termination of pregnancy should be considered if rubella in early pregnancy is confirmed. *Bacteriuria* has been associated with preterm labour. There is, as yet, no recommended routine screening for other infections associated with adverse infant or neonatal outcomes.

Drugs in pregnancy should be avoided unless absolutely essential, because of potential teratogenic effects. Drugs for epilepsy are known to be associated with congenital abnormalities and epileptic therapy needs to be carefully reviewed on an individual basis. Pregnant women should be warned against self-medication (including over-the-counter purchases), illegal drugs (such as heroin, cocaine and marijuana) and social drugs such as tobacco and alcohol, an established cause of embryopathy.

Smoking and subsequent respiratory diseases. There is evidence that young children whose mothers smoked during pregnancy have more respiratory illness during their first two or three years of life. The influence of smoking exposure during pregnancy may be even more damaging than passive exposure to smoke after birth.[18] Prevention begins before pregnancy.

Primary prevention in early life

Nutrition. Human milk is the optimum human infant food. However, specific *health* benefits are difficult to confirm in westernised societies as breast-feeding mothers tend also to be socially advantaged. Bottle-fed babies have a greater likelihood of respiratory and other illnesses mainly because of environmental disadvantage such as smoking by their mothers.[19] Breast milk may provide optimum nutrients for brain growth; there is evidence that children who were breast fed are more intelligent than bottle-fed babies.[20] Recent evidence linking low weight at one year with subsequent risk of coronary heart disease[21] provides further evidence of the importance of optimal nutrition in infancy.

Avoidance of *unsuitable diets* in infancy can prevent morbidity. Undiluted cow's milk may cause hypocalcaemic convulsions in the newborn. High solute infant milks can cause dangerous hypernatraemic dehydration during gastroenteritis. Goat's milk contains very low folic acid levels and is usually unpasteurised. The soya milks may not provide sufficient protein and have recently been shown to have high aluminium levels, a possible risk factor for Alzheimer's disease.

'Allergic' disorders, eg eczema, asthma and hayfever, are not obviously affected by the type of milk fed to a baby; breast and bottle fed babies have similar risk.[22] However *maternal* diet, avoiding allergens during pregnancy, may reduce the subsequent likelihood of allergic disorder in the child,[23] as may delay in introducing solids to the infant until at least 4 months of age.

Vitamin deficiency. Vitamin supplementation is necessary to prevent scurvy and rickets in artificially fed infants. Some breast fed babies, eg those born to mothers with marginal vitamin D status, also need supplements. Standard infant milk formulas provide adequate amounts of vitamins A and D, and oversupplementation should be avoided. In older children, a balanced diet containing recommended levels of vitamins and other essential nutrients provides normal growth and development.

Immunisations against diphtheria, tetanus, whooping cough, measles, mumps, rubella and poliomyelitis are effective primary preventive procedures and their administration should be given according to the routine schedules and not delayed (see Chapter 7). *Elimination* of these diseases from a population by immunisation programmes requires higher levels of uptake than those currently recommended. To achieve such levels a more positive approach to immunisation is likely to be necessary with all children being immunised unless there are strong parental objections or valid contraindications. Immunisation before entry to nursery classes or primary school seems essential. BCG immunisation in the newborn period, if properly administered, prevents miliary TB in vulnerable infants and is given to children of families at risk of tuberculosis.

Secondary prevention in early life

Neonatal screening

Biochemical. The Guthrie test, on blood routinely collected at 7–10 days after birth, detects pre-symptomatic *phenylketonuria* and can be combined with tests for other aminoacid disorders and *hypothyroidism*. Early diagnosis and treatment following this secondary preventive procedure can prevent brain or other damage in these conditions. Screening for haemoglobinopathies in the newborn period, eg *sickle cell disease*, is feasible but is only carried out in the UK at present in high risk areas. Perhaps 90% of babies with cystic fibrosis could be identified by examining for high levels of serum immuno-reactive trypsin but this test is not undertaken in the UK. The benefit of early diagnosis is not definite for either cystic fibrosis or sickle cell disease as neither fulfils all the generally accepted criteria for screening,[24] particularly the requirement that there is a really effective treatment. The possibility of future improvements in management could well alter the situation.

Neonatal examination. Clinical screening for *congenital dislocation of the hip* is generally recommended; however the incidence of late diagnosed CDH may not have been reduced.[25] Ultrasound examination of the neonatal hip may prove more reliable than clinical examination. All newborn babies are recommended to have a *general physical examination* before discharge from the maternity unit. Identification of cataracts, with early surgery, may prevent blindness. Obvious external congenital abnormalities are usually noticed by the mother but congenital heart disease or other internal abnormalities may be detected by routine examination, providing an opportunity for secondary prevention.

Preschool developmental surveillance

Preschool development surveillance is receiving considerable attention with the increasing involvement of general practitioners in the work and the recent publication of two reports,[4,26] which have demonstrated gaps in our understanding of many current preventive practices, especially child surveillance.

Parents are becoming increasingly involved in the early recognition and management of many childhood disorders, especially those detected in community child health surveillance programmes. This should provide earlier identification and better acceptance of problems with improved outcome for the child and family.

Evaluation of current procedures, many of which are of doubtful or unproven benefit, is a priority area for research. The resource implications of routine surveillance are large and are likely to increase with the recent government proposals that general practice should take over the bulk of this work. A strong second-tier community child health service will be needed to provide specialised assessment and advice for problems identified at the primary level and secondary preventive management of children with severe or complex disorders.

Special sense screening

Severe sensori-neural deafness (ie greater than 55 decibels hearing loss in the better ear) needs to be detected as early as possible if it is accepted that early intervention, including the provision of hearing aids, is necessary to provide the maximal opportunity for effective communication. The *distraction test* commonly performed at 7 or 8 months may not be an adequate method for detecting hearing loss and requires further evaluation. *Neonatal screening* with the auditory response cradle or other electro-physiological tests is under evaluation and may prove a more effective population screen. Parents can be involved by completing a *check list* for the detection of hearing loss, especially when there are risk factors such as a family history of deafness or specific problems in the newborn period.

Conductive deafness. Secretory otitis media (glue ear) commonly accompanies upper respiratory tract infections in early childhood and may be associated with conductive deafness. In most cases the condition resolves spontaneously. Surgery, often with the insertion of tympanostomy tubes, is frequently undertaken to prevent speech and language delay which may be associated with the deafness, but there is no good evidence from randomised control trials to support its widespread use. Indeed, some studies have shown long-term damage to the eardrum and deafness resulting from the operative intervention. Speech and language problems are more common in disadvantaged families as are respiratory infections which may be associated with 'glue-ear'. It is presently unclear whether the hearing impairment, which is usually temporary, or the social circumstances is more relevant.

Vision screening. The early identification and treatment of severe visual defects may prevent amblyopia. A fixed *squint* detected at any age should be referred for ophthalmological assessment as should any squint persisting after the age of 3 months.

Undescended testes

Boys with undescended testes, ie testes not descended normally, and all ectopic testes need referral to a specialist. The risk of infertility and malignancy may be reduced with properly positioned testes.

Emotional and behavioural disturbance

Emotional and behavioural disturbance in early life may be associated with various risk factors including isolation of the mother and maternal depression.[27] Lead toxicity from environmental lead in dust and water is also a recognised cause of disordered thinking and impaired impulse control in early life. Increasing recognition of this problem has led to the level for defining lead toxicity being lowered to an upper blood level of 1.2 μmol/l. It has been shown that the effect of lead is independent of the numerous social disadvantages to children living in high lead environments,[28] but the fact that these environments so often coincide with poor housing and other indices of deprivation adds further weight to the priority for improving social conditions. *Speech and language delay* is associated with lack of stimulation in the home. Preventive interventions include the provision of opportunities for social interaction and support and the enrichment of the child's experience with early enhanced input. Other *developmental problems* often relate to social disadvantage. Enhanced pre-school educational experience, for example the 'head start' programme in the USA, may prevent continuing problems.

The early identification of neuro-developmental problems may improve outcome. The *1981 Education Act* requires that 50% of children who will subsequently have special educational needs should be identified, often by the health services, by the age of 1 year and 80% by the age of 2 years. This may not prove realistic in practice but in theory may reduce disability and prevent handicap by comprehensive assessment and an individualised programme of care. The Children Act (1989) may facilitate these activities.

'*Targeting*' of health resources and personnel by identifying socioeconomic or environmental *risk factors* in families is widely recommended for the prevention of *child abuse* and *SIDS* but there is little evidence to justify this practice. Up to 70% of the total population may be 'targeted'; up to 40% of subsequently identified cases will be missed. Most of the identified risk factors appear to influence relative rather than absolute risk. Improved understanding of the underlying causes is required for prevention of such disorders.

Prevention of death in childhood after the first year

Many deaths after the first year of life are preventable; accidents are the most common cause (see also Chapter 8), and there are marked social class associations. Respiratory deaths remain important and suicide among older children is increasing. Figure 10.8 shows the proportions of deaths from different causes in children aged 1–4 and 5–14 years.

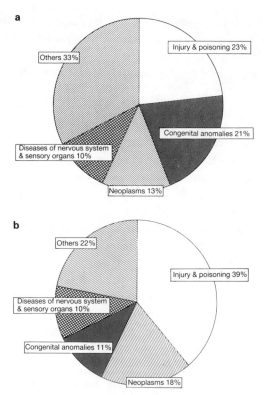

Fig. 10.9 *Distribution of major causes of deaths in children, England and Wales 1989.* **a**, *age 1–4 years;* **b**, *5–14 years.* Source: *OPCS.*

Prevention during the school years

Medical examination on school entry may identify previously undetected physical abnormalities, leading to interventions which might prevent disability or handicap. Systematic *review of (adequate) records* may confirm that all is well without formal physical examination. Advances in local, regional and national child health computing systems should facilitate the ready availability of useful records to provide evidence of previous concern or problems and the child's immunisation and surveillance record. *Parent-held records* are being evaluated in many districts as a supplement to the computer-held summary. Better records and computer systems with improved data are required for clinical service provision, for management purposes, for evaluation of process and outcome, and for epidemiological purposes to improve understanding of the factors which underlie ill-health and less than optimal development in childhood.

Continuing *surveillance of growth* throughout the early school years may help identify a few children with unsuspected physical problems including growth hormone deficiency. Regular growth measurement is probably useful for monitoring children who have been abused and who are on child protection registers. Failure of such children to grow normally suggests that the social intervention provided is not adequate.

Vision screening at school entry and every subsequent three years will detect remediable visual defects, especially acquired myopia, and so prevent visual handicap. Screening for colour blindness in boys at about eleven years may prevent inappropriate career choices.

Educational assessment, appropriate placement and/or support, including health service input, may prevent handicap in children with educational special needs such as *learning difficulties*. *Specific learning disabilities* including 'dyslexia' often have definable physical associations such as attention deficit disorder, clumsiness and hyperactivity. Accurate identification of such problems leading to individualised programmes of classroom and home care may prevent handicap, and may reduce the likelihood of the child becoming an 'educational failure', with the increased risk of social alienation, and later criminal behaviour. Any child with an educational problem requires an expert medical assessment.

Deafness in the population might be reduced by turning down the volume at pop-concerts and the presently fashionable portable stereos.

Prevention during adolescence

Adolescence is a time of experimentation: adolescents have the right to make mistakes but should be prevented as far as possible from making lethal mistakes. A disconcerting 30% of 16-year-old girls regularly smoke cigarettes[29] indicating a gross failure of preventive health education (see Chapter 2).

Health education in schools may reduce sexual problems and substance abuse including drugs and alcohol. Like recommendations for *physical exercise* and a *healthy diet*, this is probably a 'best bet' rather than a proven preventive procedure. For school children, school-based health education initiatives integrated into different parts of the curriculum appear most effective in reinforcing messages appropriate to the development of the child throughout the school years, with the core aim of promoting self esteem for developing and practising effective life skills. Promising results have been shown in preventing children from starting smoking.[30]

Avoidance of *adolescent pregnancy*, which is associated with adverse outcome both for mothers and babies, especially when the mother is under 18 years, should be included in the school health curriculum. *Preparation for parenthood* is a necessary part of training to be a good citizen.

Accidents are a major cause of death in childhood with *road-traffic deaths* particularly important in teenage males. Alcohol is known to be a critical factor in these deaths. Legislation to improve safety[31] is evidently an effective way of preventing accidents. The likely association between television and *violence* has preventive implications. Alienation can be a problem in teenagers and may be a factor in *adolescent suicide.*

Drug abuse may be amenable to prevention through education, although environmental disincentives, such as restrictions on sales to potential abusers, may be more effective. Health education in schools to avoid unhealthy behaviours such as smoking, alcohol, solvent and drug abuse, is primarily aimed at increasing self esteem. However, evaluation of the efficacy of these current approaches to prevention is required.

Adult implications of paediatric disorder

Although a great deal is known about risk factors in adult conditions like coronary heart disease, and considerable energy has been directed to the prevention of premature mortality in adults, there is still a paucity of information about the origins and possibilities for prevention of adult disease in childhood.

Blood pressure. Although many children with high blood pressure have associated renal or cardiovascular problems, essential hypertension does occur in childhood and its prevalence increases with age. There is evidence that tracking of blood pressure begins early in life. Low birthweight, especially low birthweight in association with a comparatively large placenta, appears to be an important determinant of subsequent high blood pressure. Certain interventions associated with dietary manipulation in early life, such as lower salt or drug therapy for essential hypertension, may prevent subsequent associated morbidity. Routine blood pressure screening is not recommended at present before adolescence although individual children may benefit if hypertension is identified when blood pressure is measured, while they are being examined for some medical reason.

Coronary artery disease prevention in childhood remains a theoretical possibility except in cases of familial hypercholesterolaemia when dietary manipulation associated with lowering of plasma cholesterol may postpone disease. Differing patterns of diet between different populations who have differing rates of coronary artery disease in adulthood suggest the possibility of prevention through dietary means.

Obesity. Fat babies may become fat children but the majority of fat adults were *not* fat children.[32] There is conflicting evidence about the relationship of obesity in childhood to adult cardiovascular disease (see Chapter 5). Although there may be benefits to populations from 'healthier' diets, there is little evidence that detecting and treating individual obese children is beneficial.

Behavioural disorder. Family disruption in early life (potentially preventable) has been shown to increase the relative risk of depression in adult life, suicide in females and chronic bowel problems in adult males.

Child sexual abuse, more commonly recognised in females, may predispose to depression in adult life, feeding disorders or other psychological and social problems.

General preventive implications for adult ill-health

Improvements in morbidity have been achieved through community preventive health programmes aimed at changes in life-styles including eating a healthier diet, smoking less, drinking less alcohol and taking regular exercise. These programmes have been directed at adults, but health related behaviour, patterns and attitudes to food, exercise and smoking are acquired and established in childhood, and it is well known that established habits are difficult to break. Therefore, for the maximum impact it would seem most effective to introduce a preventive approach at the earliest possible age. There has been recent concern about the low levels of physical exercise undertaken by most children in the UK and the effect that this may have on the future health of their hearts.

Although specific medical interventions in childhood may help prevent later illness, the pervasive influence of social disadvantage on health and development is the priority area for intervention. A healthy child population will result in a healthy adult population. Individuals should be provided with the opportunities to achieve their potential in health, in education and in work. Unfulfilled potential and lost opportunity due to social or environmental disadvantage in childhood is a strange waste of resources in a rich country like the UK. A change in the allocation of resources, associated with an increased political commitment to the needs of children, especially those children from disadvantaged backgrounds and those with special needs, would prevent much ill health.

CONCLUSIONS AND RECOMMENDATIONS

1 *Immunisation programmes* should be supported and uptake improved, particularly in the deprived social groups.

2 *'Parenting skills'* should be promoted, especially in deprived areas, through schools, antenatal classes and parents' groups.

3 *Training* for child health workers and others involved with child care should be improved to include the early detection of problems in childhood and of families vulnerable because of their social circumstances.

4 More *research* into the effectiveness and cost-effectiveness of current pre-school and school health *surveillance programmes* should be undertaken.

5 Investment in and development of child health computing and related *information systems* should be increased to provide better data, with a view to effective prevention.

6 The delivery of *health education/promotion programmes* through rigorous evaluation should be improved with particular emphasis on programmes directed at school children. Such programmes should include attention to diet and exercise.

7 Further measures to *reduce accidents and smoking* in individuals and in communities should be developed.

8 *Integration* of the various *services* involved with child health care should be improved to avoid gaps in provision and to ensure optimal uptake, especially for children with special health care needs and those from disadvantaged backgrounds.

9 Governmental review of, and *action on*, social inequalities related to health should be encouraged.

10 Increased (political) commitment to recognising and meeting the *needs of children and families* should be promoted.

11 Later life

The various social definitions of 'old age' as starting at age 65 or 75 or at the time of compulsory retirement have no biological validity. Ageing in the sense of senescence is characterised by a decline over time in an individual's ability to respond adaptively to challenges from the external or internal environment. Examples of such challenges include an infection such as influenza, an unexpected stumble while walking, thrombosis in an artery, a malignant clone of cells or an ill-considered dose of some drug prescribed by a doctor. Ageing as a biological process is therefore characterised by an increase with age in the risk of death. In the human this rise starts around the age of 13 and with minor perturbations in early adult life the risk of death increases smoothly, continuously and approximately exponentially with age (Fig. 11.1). There is no discontinuity in later life in terms of risk of death, prevalence of chronic disease, use of health services or ability to respond to treatment that can justify separation of 'the elderly' from the rest of the human race. Old age begins biologically at the age of 13, and the preventive medicine of old age must be seen as a lifelong process. In this sense the topics considered in other chapters in this report are as

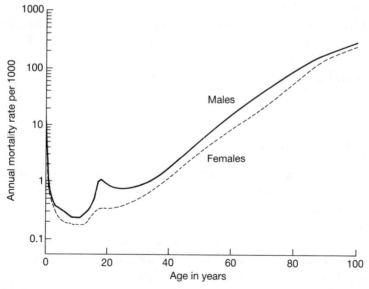

Fig. 11.1 *Age and sex-specific annual mortality rates, England and Wales, 1980–82.* Source: *OPCS.*

relevant to health in later life as they are to younger ages. In this chapter we restrict consideration to aspects of preventive medicine as applied to people in the sixth decade of life and beyond, merely to avoid repetition and not because of any fundamental difference between younger and older citizens.

Expectation of life at birth in England and Wales has passed 71 years for men and 77 years for women. At least 74% of men and 84% of women will reach the age of 65 and 46% of men and 66% of women the age of 75. Old age is therefore a time of life that most of us will experience and all of us should plan for.

Optimal ageing

It has been traditional in medical teaching to try to distinguish between 'normal ageing' and 'disease'. This approach is intellectually flawed and undesirable in practice. The word 'normal' has at least three different meanings which are too easily confused. It may mean 'common', it may mean 'healthy' or it may mean 'having statistical properties associated with the name of Gauss'. Unfortunately, what is common is not necessarily healthy and few biological variables actually have Gaussian properties if examined critically. Similarly, 'disease' has no generally agreed definition but the word carries the implication that something that is labelled 'disease' is a proper concern of doctors and a cause for sympathy and support from others, while something that has been labelled 'normal' is not.[1] In practice, if an old person is facing difficulty or discomfort the question to be asked is not: 'is this normal ageing or disease?', but rather: 'what can be done to help?' The same question needs to be the basis of preventive medicine for later life. We should be concerned not with 'normal' ageing but with optimal ageing.

Intrinsic and extrinsic ageing

The decrements in structure and function that lead to the characteristic loss of biological fitness with age arise from the interaction between intrinsic (genetic) and extrinsic (environmental and lifestyle) factors.[2] In very broad terms our genetic endowment determines the maximum lifespan we could hope to obtain, while extrinsic factors determine how close we actually approach it. What disabilities we accumulate on the way will have both intrinsic and extrinsic determinants, and how well we are able to cope with such disabilities will depend on our social resources including money, housing and family or other human support, and thus the severity of environmental challenge. Preventive care in later life must concern itself with more than medical matters.

The scope of prevention

The aim of prevention for later life is to reduce the incidence of disability. Preventive modification of intrinsic ageing will not be feasible until the biochemical processes involved in the genetic determinants of ageing are understood. While there are likely to be important advances in this field in the next two or three decades, for the time being prevention of age-associated disability will be dependent on modification of extrinsic ageing and on reducing environmental challenge. Until recently, health and social services policy has been dominated by the latter as far as action for people in later life has been concerned. One reason for this has been the assumption that the effects of extrinsic factors will necessarily be cumulative and that reduction of plasma cholesterol, say, in old age will have a negligible effect on the total lifetime accumulation of cholesterol in a person's arteries. While, undoubtedly, some determinants of health and disability in old age are active early in life (the amount of bone tissue laid down at adolescence is one) the scope for prevention in later life is properly a subject for empirical experiment not for armchair theorising. This needs to be more widely recognised; trials of preventive medicine commonly exclude people aged over 70 on the untested assumption that they would not be able to benefit. Not surprisingly, therefore, there is a dearth of good studies of preventive interventions in later life.

Observational studies, for example that of Alameda County California,[3] imply that healthy lifestyles are associated with lower death rates in the old as in the young. The Alameda County study examined the association of health-related practices (no cigarettes, moderate alcohol intake, regular exercise, controlled body weight and regular sleeping hours). Subjects aged over 70 years with four or five of these factors had a lower mortality (35% lower over 9 years for men and 22% for women) than did subjects with two or less. Clearly, what observational studies of this kind cannot prove is whether these practices themselves could reduce mortality if started for the first time in old age, or whether they are merely markers of previous good health and lifestyle. In terms of good advice to an ageing population we can for the time being do no better than to follow the precept of Henry Acland in 1854:[4]

> In a scientific sense, parts of the only available evidence of an enquiry like this are necessarily inconclusive: much of the useful business of life would come to an end, and the physician would throw away many lives, if he could not, or would not, manfully act upon the greater probability.

In other words, the health-related practices of Alameda County make good sense.

The present and future of old age

Life expectancy is increasing in Britain in old age as at younger, but we have no adequate data in Britain to tell us whether health in old age is improving or deteriorating. American optimists such as Fries[5] believe that we are living longer because we are fitter and that when we do die it will be because we have reached our intrinsic maximum and we will die rapidly and without a prolonged period of dependency. Others fear that much of the recent average increase in longevity in later life has come about not because of improved health but because of improved survival of the ill and disabled.[6] At present we simply do not know which of these two contrasting views is correct, and many gerontologists suspect that both processes are at work.

The incidence of many diseases increases with age, but typically the case-fatality also rises; in other words, the older we are the more likely we are to develop a disease but also the sooner we will die from it. In general therefore the age-specific prevalence of most conditions does not rise as steeply as one might expect from incidence rates. In terms of numbers of individuals affected, the ageing of the population in Britain and other countries will therefore in general have a greater effect on the need for acute care of incident disease than on the chronic care of prevalent disease. Tragically one exception to this general conclusion lies with Alzheimer's type of dementia. The later the onset of this disease the slower its progression, and the survival time of patients with dementia is increasing, probably owing to improvements in nursing care. We can therefore expect a disproportionate increase in the numbers of people afflicted with dementia in the next decade. This will create a corresponding increase in the need for various types of institutional care since the scope for humane domiciliary care of demented people is more limited than for people with physical disabilities.

The pattern of disease will also be determined by changes in incidence and survival. For example, as noted elsewhere in this report, the incidence of stroke seems to be falling while that of proximal femoral fracture is rising. The future prevalence of disability in old age therefore remains uncertain, but some fears are inevitable that preventive medicine in later life, by prolonging survival, may increase the total sum of human misery rather than reducing it. One approach to assessing the implications of survival is to use a Life Table approach to measure not just life expectancy at different ages but also active or independent life expectancy, that is to say years of life without the need of help from

Table 11.1   Life expectancy in years; Massachusetts, 1974

| | Men | | | Women | | |
Age	Total	Active	Dependent	Total	Active	Dependent
65–69	13.1	9.3	3.8	19.5	10.6	8.9
70–74	11.9	8.2	3.7	15.9	8.0	7.9
75–79	9.6	6.5	3.1	13.2	7.1	6.1
80–84	8.2	4.8	3.4	9.8	4.8	5.0
85–	6.5	3.3	3.2	7.7	2.8	4.9

Source: Katz *et al.*, 1983.[7]

others in performing the basic activities of daily living (Table 11.1). At present there are no good data on active life expectancy from Britain (and we ought to be setting up some national system for obtaining them) but the Table presents figures from Massachusetts.[7] Two issues of interest emerge from this Table:

1. The number of years of dependency to be expected diminishes with increasing age at baseline (columns 3 and 6). In other words, the longer that one can preserve health and prevent disability into old age the fewer years of ultimate dependency one can expect. While bearing in mind that the data are American and not British they suggest that successful prevention, in the sense of delaying the onset of disabling disease, will reduce overall dependency rather than increasing it.

2. The Table reveals the less reassuring fact that although women outlive men on average (columns 1 and 4), as is universal in economically advanced nations, their extra years of life are entirely accounted for by years of dependency (columns 3 and 6). From what is known of dependency in old age this is unlikely to be attributable to specific disease entities. Rather it is more likely to be a manifestation of generally lower physical functional reserves in women compared with men, particularly in terms of muscle bulk and strength. Thus any disease-related disability in an old woman is more likely to reduce her function below the threshold of independence than would be the case for a man. The male–female difference in muscle bulk and strength is to a large extent genetic, reflecting the evolutionary history of our species, but in addition will be due to different patterns of physical activity during both childhood and adult life. The Table suggests that this is an area requiring research but that in the meantime an educational system that assumes that

young women should be less physically active than men should be questioned.

SPECIFIC ASPECTS OF PREVENTIVE MEDICINE IN LATER LIFE

Cardiovascular disease (see also Chapter 5)

Cardiovascular disease accounts for a large proportion of disability and more than half the deaths in later life, particularly among men. Recent studies have shown the benefits of control of high blood pressure at ages at least up to 80,[8,9] and studies of subjects above that age are needed in view of the importance of stroke as a cause of disability. While the controlled trials indicate the benefit of treatment under the selection procedures and quality of clinics involved, it is not yet clear what the cost-benefit balance will be of screening programmes for hypertension among elderly patients in British general practice. This uncertainty raises both ethical and economic problems. It could be argued that it would be sensible for the elderly person who is aware of the risks of side-effects of the relevant drugs, and prepared to undertake the necessary levels of surveillance of treatment, to seek blood pressure measurement and control. By so doing the subject could be regarded as identifying him- or herself as a member of the population to which the original controlled trials were applicable. On the other hand it could be argued that it would be—or at least could be seen as— inequitable and uneconomic for some people to be able to demand, at public expense, care that is not offered to all. Perhaps the answer is to recognise an ethical obligation on Government and professions to carry out the necessary controlled trials and on the public to participate in them.

Cholesterol

In early and mid-adult life, blood lipids are powerful indicators of the risk of coronary heart disease, and control of plasma cholesterol has long been advocated in these age groups. Older age groups have in general been excluded from these recommendations, chiefly because plasma cholesterol has often not emerged as a risk factor for ischaemic heart disease in later life, particularly in the earlier epidemiological studies, and partly, as suggested above because of perhaps incomplete models of the mechanisms linking cholesterol in the blood to atheroma in the arterial wall. In more recent studies in the USA, serum lipids are emerging as predictors of ischaemic heart disease at later ages than in earlier studies, perhaps because extrinsic ageing processes and differential survival effects have been changing in successive cohorts of the middle-aged and elderly. Furthermore, evaluation of the epidemiology and interventive trials linking plasma cholesterol to ischaemic heart disease indicate that lowering cholesterol has a more rapid effect on the incidence of the disease than seems to be compatible with an effect through reduction on the cumulative lifetime 'dosage' of plasma cholesterol.[10] This implies that a larger benefit from control of cholesterol in old age may be expected than was at one time assumed.

While no firm recommendations can be made at this stage, there is a clear need for randomised controlled trials of cholesterol reduction to be extended into later age groups, and in the meantime it would be sensible for older people to adopt a 'prudent diet' of reduced total fat and increased polyunsaturated/saturated fat ratio (see Chapters 3 and 4).

Cigarette smoking

Cigarette smoking is a further risk factor that has been attacked less consistently in later life than in younger age groups on the often tacit assumption that it will already have done any harm it is going to do. In two North American studies[11,12] it has emerged that older people with coronary disease who give up smoking do better than those who do not. Clearly, it is never too late to give up cigarette smoking and older people and their medical advisers should strive to bring this about.

Strokes

Apart from high blood pressure, one of the consistent risk factors for stroke in later life is the presence of atrial fibrillation, and approximately 5% of men and 3% of women aged over 65 years are in atrial fibrillation in the British population.[13] In British people in this age group with established fibrillation there is an approximately three- to four-fold increased risk of stroke compared with people of matched age and sex,[14] and higher risk ratios have been reported from the USA. It has also been shown that subjects with atrial fibrillation have a higher prevalence of 'silent' cerebral infarcts than is found in non-fibrillating controls.[14] These findings might imply that a proportion of the excess strokes in the presence of fibrillation are due to emboli and therefore susceptible to anticoagulant therapy, but on the other hand atrial fibrillation might simply be a 'marker' for generalised vascular disease including the cerebral circulation. The Framingham study[15] suggested that stroke is a particularly high risk early in the onset of atrial fibrillation. Clinically, established fibrillation may be preceded by a phase of recurrent fibrillation during which the risk of stroke may be high in an elderly person, although a study of paroxysmal fibrillation in young life assurance applicants did not find this.[16]

Recent trials[17] indicate that anticoagulant therapy can greatly reduce the risk of stroke in people with atrial fibrillation. Moreover, this reduction can be achieved at comparatively low levels of anticoagulation and the benefit greatly outweighs the risk of side-effects such as bleeding. It is sometimes claimed that elderly people are particularly susceptible to the ill effects of anticoagulant therapy but provided that selection and supervision are adequate this is probably not the case.[18] In brief, the evidence indicates that doctors should give serious consideration to anticoagulant therapy in all elderly patients with atrial fibrillation for whom there are no specific contraindications.

Falls and fractures

Fractures are common among elderly people and the great majority are due to simple falls. Even without causing fractures falls can have a profound effect on the quality of life of an old person. Serious hazards such as hypothermia, pressure necrosis and rhabdomyolysis are only part of the picture. The loss of confidence and anxiety generated by falling can lead to loss of mobility (thereby perhaps increasing rather than diminishing the risk of further falls) and to reduced social contact and possibly unnecessary institutionalisation.

One of the common fractures in old age is that of the proximal femur (often referred to as fracture of the femoral neck or simply as fracture of the hip). This is a serious injury, more than a quarter of sufferers die within six months and more than half the survivors have some persistent pain or swelling of the affected leg or an increase in dependency. It is also a costly injury in terms of the use of health and social services. The fracture is becoming more common in Britain partly because there are more people living to the ages at which it occurs, but also because for reasons that are not yet clear, the risk of the fracture in old age is increasing.

In adult men, the risk of falling is fairly constant and low until the seventh decade when an exponential increase into old age occurs. In women the risk of falls is greater than in men at all ages, but they also show a circumscribed peak in risk of falling around the age of 50, which contributes to the rise in incidence of distal forearm fracture at that age.[19] Although the risk of falling increases exponentially at ages above 65 in both sexes, the risk of proximal femoral fracture increases much more steeply while the incidence of distal forearm fracture does not increase over this age range. This seems to indicate that the older a person is the more likely she is to fall but the less likely is she to throw her arm as a protective response to falling. The genesis of proximal femoral fracture seems therefore to depend on three factors: falling, bone weakness, and the protective factors of which neuromuscular responses are one.[20] Muscle bulk and subcutaneous fat may also act as more passive protection in preventing transmission of the full force of a fall to the bones.

Bone weakness

Two mains forms of bone weakness affect old people:

- *Osteomalacia*, in which bone is inadequately calcified, is due to deficiency of vitamin D, a vitamin that is obtained either from the diet or by exposure of the skin to sunlight.

- *Osteoporosis*. By far the commonest form of bone weakness in old age is osteoporosis, in which the bone is normal but greatly reduced in quantity.

We develop bone from childhood into early adult life but thereafter bone tissue is gradually reabsorbed over time. In men this loss occurs at a more or less steady rate but in women there is in addition a five-to ten-year phase of very rapid loss after the menopause. The amount, and hence the strength of our bones in old age therefore depend on the amount we laid down in early life and the rate at which we have lost it thereafter. Because girls lay down less bone than boys, and subsequently experience the rapid post-menopausal loss, osteoporosis is more common among women than among men. It is thought that the amount laid down in childhood is partly under genetic control but is also affected by the amount of physical exercise and muscular development and also by the amount of calcium in the diet. Studies in the USA suggest that on a self-chosen diet many adolescent girls consume less calcium than is desirable and that this is becoming more common. The rate of bone loss in adult life is probably retarded by physical exercise and may in some people be accelerated by dietary factors, including insufficient calcium. Cigarette smoking increases the risk of osteoporosis by a number of mechanisms, including bringing forward the age at which the menopause occurs. On average, women who smoke experience the menopause and the associated rapid bone loss up to two years earlier than non-smoking women. Osteoporosis is also more common among people who are below average weight for their height.

Significance of osteoporosis

The significance of osteoporosis in causing fractures in old age has been underestimated by some writers. If old people who have fractured their hips are compared with people of the same age who have not—the 'case-control' method of study—very often no difference is found between the two groups in the prevalence of osteoporosis. This does not mean that osteoporosis is unimportant, however. Fractures occur when the strength of bone falls below a certain level and in the British population osteoporosis is so common that all old people have bones below this level. Thus, the differences that will be found in the case-control method will be the factors that determine which old people fall and the state of their protective factors as outlined above. Nonetheless, if the bones were not weakened by osteoporosis, falling over and lack of protective factors would not cause so many fractures. Therefore osteoporosis is the important determinant of overall incidence of fractures in old age even though it may not emerge as such in case-control studies. (Technically, the problem is that of 'over-matching' in which matching cases and controls for one variable, in this case age, also matches for the causative variable one is trying to detect— osteoporosis—because the two are so closely correlated.)

In the long term, prevention of fractures in old age will therefore depend on the reduction of the prevalence of osteoporosis in the population. There is no doubt that the use of Hormone Replacement Therapy (HRT) by menopausal women will delay the onset of the rapid phase of bone loss and reduce the risk of subsequent fractures. Although HRT carries some slight risk of side-effects (see Chapter 6), this is now thought to be negligible if care is taken in the initial assessment and in the surveillance of women opting for it. Cigarette smoking is an important factor, and some consider that it may be responsible for the increase in risk of proximal femoral fracture over recent decades. As for life style, although the evidence is not yet entirely firm, it is prudent to aim for an average body weight, an adequate calcium content in the diet and regular physical exercise. These factors are probably most important during childhood and adolescence but are sensible lifelong habits.

Prevention of falls

In the short term, the main approaches to prevention of proximal femoral fracture will lie with preventing falls and addressing factors that determine whether a fall will result in a fracture. Many falls by elderly people are due to apparently preventable hazards such as loose rugs or poor lighting and there is increasing evidence that poor design in the environment, particularly ill-designed and visually confusing stairways may have an important influence.[21] As we grow older we become more dependent on vision than on information from muscles, tendons and joints in avoiding falls, and our vision often deteriorates. More attention should be given by architects and urban planners to the implications of visual problems common in an ageing population.

Drugs and falling

An association between prescribed drugs and falling by old people is a consistent feature of studies in Britain and the USA. Long-acting hypnotics, tranquillisers and antidepressants seem to be particularly dangerous and there is little doubt that these are overprescribed for elderly people. Most benzodiazepines have a longer action on the central nervous system of old people than the manufacturers claim and can, and probably should, be avoided as hypnotics. In contrast with some studies in other countries, alcohol does not seem to be a numerically important cause of falls among British elderly people (see page 115), although it clearly contributes in some individual cases.

Exercise

There are several reasons for believing that regular physical exercise can prevent both falls and fractures among older people. As already noted, exercise can retard the rate of age-associated bone loss and it will also maintain muscle bulk and strength. Daily and frequent movements of the limbs will also reduce the physical stiffness of joints and increase the range of joint movement. Less clear is whether regular exercise will foster neuromuscular co-ordination and thus both reduce the risk of falling and improve the protective response to a fall, although there is some reported evidence that this may be so and further studies are in progress.[22]

Screening and case finding

The Government has recently introduced annual assessment of people aged 75 years and over as a contractual obligation of general practitioners, but there is some uncertainty at present about the best way of ensuring that this will achieve useful results. With a few praiseworthy exceptions, trials of screening and case-finding among the elderly patients in general practice have been uncontrolled or non-randomised. It is to be hoped that comparative trials of different processes of assessment will be carried out in the next few years to identify the most effective.

British approaches to screening and case-finding in later life have tended to focus on standardised functional assessments, for example in activities of daily living, eyesight and hearing. In North America there is more enthusiasm for screening for asymptomatic disease. Medical recommendations there include regular breast, rectal and pelvic examination, mammography, faecal occult blood and blood pressure measurement, and a number of biochemical tests on blood samples.[23] None of these has yet undergone rigorous evaluation in a British elderly population, and in our view should only be introduced in the context of a formal experimental trial.

The common assumption that case-finding will inevitably be effective is derived from some studies which discovered large amounts of morbidity among elderly patients that was previously unknown to their general practitioners. Not all studies have found this, and given that at least 70% of people aged 65 and over are in contact with their general practice in the course of a year, the undiscovered morbidity may be a reflection on the failure of some general practitioners to make best use of normal consultations.

Surveillance

Two controlled trials found that surveillance led to an increase in hospital admissions but a reduction in total days in institutions among the visited elderly people compared with the controls. Whether this occurred because a better database held in general practice facilitated early discharge from hospital or because a 'backlog' of hitherto unrecognised pathology was referred for treatment at an earlier stage when it is more rapidly treatable remains unclear. Also unclear is whether the differences between the surveillance group and the controls would persist after the first 'sweep'.

Social contact

Reviewing the studies as a whole, it seems that the routine assessment of the functional disabilities and needs of vulnerable elderly people may lead to a reduction in mortality. The mechanisms of this effect are uncertain and may be related not so much to the actual treatments or interventions offered as to the well-established but little understood phenomenon that old people with an established 'social network' of friends and social contacts survive better than those who are isolated and friendless.[24]

Sensory function

Among the specific requirements of the new general practitioner contract is the annual assessment of sensory function of patients aged 75 years and over. Failing vision and hearing are common in later life and may contribute to social isolation. Visually impaired old people may be fearful of going out of doors, and those with auditory impairment may find conversation difficult and embarrassing. Both impairments can restrict opportunities for mental stimulation from the media and further distance an old person from the outside world. Moreover, as already noted, both impairments restrict a person's ability to notice and avoid hazards, thus increasing the risk of accidents.

The effects of glaucoma and cataract can be improved by appropriate treatment but these diseases account for only a proportion of visual difficulties among elderly people. Age-associated changes, for example in the ability of the eye to detect contrast or to adapt to low light levels play an important role. Prevention of visual handicap in later life is therefore greatly dependent on the provision of magnifying glasses and increased lighting.

Similarly, although part of the age-associated hearing loss, universal in the population, is due to lifelong exposure to potentially reducible environmental noise, it is irreversible once established. The mainstay of preventing social handicap from deafness remains the provision of hearing aids. These are difficult to use, and care must be taken to teach the wearer how to adjust the aid for different purposes and different levels of ambient sound. Several sessions with a well-trained hearing aid technician may be required and an old person may need active encouragement to persist with the aid.

The need for rehabilitation

Two of the specific manifestations of loss of adaptability with ageing is that older people have lower levels of functional reserve and take longer to recover from illness or injury. In practice, this means that older people need specific rehabilitation after an illness or injury and if this is not provided there is a higher risk of delayed or even failed recovery of premorbid levels of function. A programme of physical rehabilitation needs to be combined, if the illness had been at all prolonged, with attention to nutrition to bring body weight and lean body mass back to desirable levels. While many elderly people, perhaps with support and encouragement from their families, can do this for themselves, some will require help from the health and social services. It is important that an older person who has lost function after a temporary illness should be persuaded to undertake rehabilitation rather than simply be given a home help or some other social prosthesis, since this will merely make lower levels of activity and further decline inevitable. As the discussion above suggests, rehabilitation following a fall should often aim to increase the physical fitness of the victim to better than premorbid levels.

Cold

As is well known, older people are more sensitive to the deleterious effects of cold (and of heat, though that is less of a British problem at present). The incidence of frank hypothermia is very low in Britain, but there is a much more important effect of cold weather in increasing mortality from vascular and infective diseases among elderly people. The processes whereby cold causes this increase in mortality, which is larger than is seen in several other countries with greater seasonal differences in temperature, remains obscure. A number of workers have suggested that it has less to do with cold itself than with the variation in temperature to which the British way of life, and more important the British way of heating, exposes elderly people.

The issue has some important implications; at present we do not know whether to recommend that an old person should keep as far as possible to one warm room in her house which may increase her exposure to chill on moving around the house, or to advise maintaining all the rooms in regular use, especially the bedroom, at a more moderate temperature. This approach could maintain heating costs at the same level but would reduce the variation in chill exposure. An additional benefit might be the encouragement to an older person to be more physically active by reducing the unpleasantness of moving from one warm room. Until further research is done this question must remain open, but either approach will require that old people can afford heating bills.

Nutrition

Surveys carried out in Britain twenty years ago suggested that there was little overt malnutrition among elderly people unless some predisposing factor in the form of physical or mental ill-health was present. There has been concern since that some more subtle effects of malnutrition on the health of older people may have been overlooked in such surveys. For example, elderly people who are chronically undernourished with thin layers of subcutaneous fat may be at higher than average risk of minor degrees of hypothermia that predispose to falls, or increase the risk of hypothermia after a fall or fracture has occurred.[25] There is also evidence that old people who have gone without food for a fairly short period, say a day, may have impaired ability to mount an adequate response to a cold environment.

Vitamin D

The relationship of vitamin D status to osteoporosis and femoral fracture may also need further evaluation. In the early 1970s frank nutritional osteomalacia was not uncommon on Tyneside, and this disappeared over a decade when the intake of vitamin D from fortified margarines was increasing among the elderly of Britain.[26] Reduction in atmospheric pollution and so less screening out of the ultraviolet radiation that produces vitamin D in the skin may also have contributed. Other studies in the 1970s showed that in Northern and Welsh settings the prevalence of histological osteomalacia in patients with proximal femoral fracture was of the order of 20–30%. Vitamin D deficiency might be related to proximal femoral fracture in several ways. It might cause bone weakness directly or it might lead to falls through proximal myopathy. On the other hand it might simply be a marker of lack of sunlight exposure due to an older person's housebound status which in turn is related to immobility and risk of falling. There is also a possibility that subclinical vitamin D deficiency may contribute in the long term to osteoporosis by causing a seasonal increase in parathyroid hormone secretion and recurrent bone attrition.[27] It has been suggested that a desirable level of vitamin D would be that which is sufficient to abolish seasonal variation, a level of intake higher than necessary merely to prevent overt osteomalacia.

At present the question of the adequacy of vitamin D intake by the elderly people of Britain is unclear. It seems likely that a proportion of older people may have less than optimal intakes, and that this proportion may be increasing as vitamin D enriched margarine in their diet is replaced by unfortified low-fat spreads. It also seems probable that EC regulations will require Britain to repeal the compulsory fortification of its margarine. If this occurs, medically supervised vitamin D supplements may prove necessary during the winter months for old people who for one reason or another have an inadequate diet and are housebound. Self-medication with vitamin D should be undertaken with care since it is poisonous in excessive doses.

As noted earlier, maintenance of body weight at or slightly above average levels is associated with good health in older people. Gross overweight can impair mobility and exacerbate osteoarthrosis of the knees but, as also implied earlier, it is not wise for old people to be underweight since this is associated with an increased risk of osteoporosis and fractures.

Self-care and defensive health care

The term 'defensive health care' was coined to designate an aspect of self-care identified as important in an American context,[28] but which may be expected to benefit old people in Britain also. It starts from the observation that older people in general receive less good care from their health and social care attendants than do younger patients. This arises partly because of the perceived 'social value' of older people compared with younger, and from often misconceived notions of the appropriateness and effectiveness of medical and social interventions in the care of older people. These in turn arise from inadequate training and education of health and social services personnel. In order to compensate for this discriminatory behaviour older people must develop their own appropriate standards of what they have a right to demand from health and social care. They should learn to recognise second-rate treatment when it is proffered to them, and learn how to use the system of care to ensure that their needs are properly catered for. They should in particular question the prescription of drugs and be more ready to request specialist opinion, and to expect active rather than palliative treatment.

The need for defensive health care may become even greater in Britain if budgetary incentives in the health system lead politicians and administrators to search for groups of the public who can be discriminated against with impunity, a role in which the politically supine British elderly have traditionally been cast. Moreover, a famous study some years ago showed that British elderly people had lower expectations of health and of their health care providers than did older people in Denmark or the USA.[29]

A determination to ensure that they obtain good quality medical and social care is only one aspect of the benefits that are likely to accrue to older people from a positive approach to their lives and worth. As noted earlier there is extensive evidence that maintaining active mental interests and social networks[24] is associated with improved well-being and health. Life is for living.

CONCLUSIONS AND RECOMMENDATIONS

1. There is increasing evidence that some preventive measures of known or probable value in younger age groups will also be beneficial to elderly people. It is never too late to give up cigarette smoking, and while the value of cholesterol reduction in later life is not yet clear, it is sensible for elderly people, as well as the young, to adopt a cholesterol-lowering diet. Careful control of high blood pressure has been shown to reduce the risk of stroke in later life as in middle age.

2. Regular physical exercise should be encouraged at all ages. Exercise slows down age-associated bone loss, helps maintain muscle bulk and strength and reduces joint stiffness, thus reducing the risk of falls and fractures. Rehabilitation after illness and injury is especially important in the elderly, and should be actively pursued.

3. Hormone replacement treatment in menopausal women also helps to reduce the risk of later fractures.

4. Careful control of the use of drugs by elderly people is especially relevant to prevention in view of the association between certain prescribed drugs and falls.

5. Atrial fibrillation is common in elderly people and is an important risk factor for stroke. Anticoagulant therapy in elderly patients with atrial fibrillation should be seriously considered.

6. More study is needed on the increase of vascular and infective illness associated with cold and on the best methods of keeping elderly people warm.

7. Annual assessment of people aged 75 and over has recently been introduced and more work is needed to ensure the best results from this policy.

8. Maintaining active mental and physical activities and social contacts is conducive to good health in elderly people. Older people should be encouraged to recognise and to expect high standards of care from medical and social services.

12 Summary and conclusions

In each of the foregoing chapters evidence has been presented on the preventability of a number of causes of morbidity and mortality. The methods by which disease may be prevented range from reducing exposure to a risk factor, through disease-specific immunisations, to screening leading to curative treatment of early disease. The priority to be accorded to each preventive activity depends on the strength of evidence of its effectiveness, the proportion of each disease which could be prevented and at what cost, and the frequency of that disease. In this final chapter we summarise various preventive activities, starting with those where the case for prevention is strongest.

Smoking

Smoking is the major risk factor for several diseases affecting people of all ages. In terms of the number of deaths attributable to smoking, ischaemic heart disease is the greatest, followed by lung cancer and chronic obstructive lung disease; it also contributes to morbidity and mortality from a number of other cancers, and to immaturity of infants born to women who smoke in pregnancy.

The evidence that these conditions could be prevented by a reduction in cigarette smoking is overwhelming. Preventive activities to reduce the number of people who smoke include legislative measures by government, promotion of non-smoking policies by local authorities, health authorities and industries, public education especially in schools, and, last but not least, advice and support from health professionals in their contacts with patients who smoke. Increasing implementation of all these activities should make a very large contribution to improving health, but further research is still needed into effective ways of helping smokers to stop and educating children not to start smoking. Detailed recommendations for action are given at the end of Chapter 2.

Infection

Despite major improvements, infections remain as important causes of mortality and morbidity, especially at the extremes of life. Many infections, notably the common viral infections of the respiratory tract, are still inaccessible to specific measures of prevention and treatment. For those preventable by immunisation, however, dramatic success can be achieved in their control, and campaigns directed at immunisation are among the most successful of public health measures. The present national policy aims at the near-universal immunisation against polio-myelitis, diphtheria, tetanus, pertussis, measles, mumps and rubella, and selective vaccination against tuberculosis.

Antibiotics have a limited but definite role in the prevention of some specific infections, for example, the prevention of meningococcal and haemophilus meningitis in close contacts, and also in the prevention of several important types of infection following surgery.

Food and water-borne infections have been greatly reduced by the provision of safe water supplies, by the development of sound practices in animal husbandry and the food industry, and by good hygienic practices in industry and the home, but recent experiences have shown how industrialised food processing can lead to problems requiring new methods of control.

Future needs in the prevention of infection include the development of vaccines against common or serious infections not yet susceptible to this form of prevention. Of the many new developments in immunisation, vaccination against meningitis caused by *Haemophilus influenzae* is soon to be introduced into the schedule for general infant immunisation.

Other important needs are continued education in the prevention of sexually transmitted disease, including AIDS, in health protection for travellers, and in sound domestic practice in food handling.

The important and common problem of hospital infection needs constant surveillance in order to ensure that known control measures are followed, and much additional study is required, especially directed at the increasing number of patients with increased vulnerability to infection.

Alcohol

The damage inflicted by alcohol is great and well documented. In addition to the well-recognised effect as a cause of liver disease, alcohol damages many other bodily systems, especially the nervous system (intoxication, black-outs, cerebrovascular accidents, permanent brain damage, peripheral neuropathy), the cardiovascular system (abnormal rhythms, high blood pressure, cardiomyopathy), and the gastrointestinal system (gastritis, pancreatitis). The relationship between alcohol consumption and road accidents is also firmly established. No less significant is the social damage inflicted by the interrelated effects of alcohol, family disruption, occupational deterioration and crime.

Strong evidence links the ill-effects of alcohol to levels of national consumption, and consumption is in its turn inversely related to the price of alcoholic drinks.

Doctors have an important role in the prevention of alcohol-related disorders by their awareness of the different manifestations of alcohol abuse, by taking a history of drinking habits, and by advising patients about safe drinking limits.

Health education should be especially directed at professionals responsible for personal care, such as health care workers, teachers and personnel officers, and at vulnerable subjects, such as children, teenagers, pregnant women, drivers and people in at-risk occupations.

In the public domain, there should be improved co-ordination of agencies with responsibility for alcohol policies. The price of alcohol should increase at least in line with inflation, and alcohol advertising should be restricted. Alcoholic drinks should carry a health warning and state their alcoholic content, although EC rules may limit the scope for Governmental action.

Although new work on the social, psychiatric and physical consequences of alcohol abuse is desirable, the main effects of this addictive agent, and many workable and effective methods of control, are well defined and need energetic implementation.

Diet

The main effects of unhealthy diets in the UK today are obesity and high levels of plasma cholesterol. More than one-third of adults are overweight and, although it is hard to quantify how much disease is attributable to this, obesity is associated with coronary heart disease, hypertension and stroke, diabetes, arthritis, and various cancers. A sensible diet therefore is one in which ideal weight is maintained. In overweight people, a reduction in calories can be achieved by cutting down on fats and sugars with a compensatory increase in fruit, vegetables and whole-grain cereals.

High plasma cholesterol levels in the UK population are associated with our high incidence of coronary heart disease. Dietary fat is the main source of plasma cholesterol, and can be reduced by a reduction of total fat consumption together with an increase in polyunsaturated fats relative to saturated fats. Experimental proof of the effect of changing diet in this way is lacking (because of the difficulty of conducting such experiments) but there is so much non-experimental evidence pointing to the efficacy of a lower fat diet that it can be recommended for the whole population, except children below the age of 5 years.

A high intake of dietary fibre is known to protect against constipation and diverticulitis, and is thought to protect against colorectal cancer; it is postulated that it may also have a protective effect against postmenopausal breast cancer and against coronary heart disease. While the extent of its effect is unknown, it is reasonable to advocate high consumption. Similarly, there is much evidence that high salt intake is associated with hypertension, and possibly also with stomach cancer. Since average UK salt consumption is greater than is physiologically required, a reduction of salt is recommended. There is evidence that cruciferous vegetables and fruit exert a protective effect against various cancers.

In summary, direct experimental evidence is not available about the protective effects which changing consumption of various dietary constituents may have, but comparisons of different populations suggest that very worthwhile reductions in cardiovascular and malignant disease could be achieved by a change in the average UK diet to one which is low in fat, sugar and salt, and high in fibre and cruciferous vegetables. Research efforts to clarify the biochemical mechanisms whereby dietary constituents lead to, or protect against, disease offer the prospect of more specific dietary advice in the future. Detailed recommendations are given at the end of Chapter 4.

Regular exercise

Lack of physical exercise is associated with coronary heart disease, obesity, osteoporosis (particularly in women), reduced muscle bulk and strength, and possibly impaired neuromuscular co-ordination in the elderly. It is not possible to quantify the reduction in incidence and mortality from coronary heart disease, other obesity-related diseases, and falls in the elderly, which could be avoided by set levels of exercise. Nevertheless, comparisons of sub-groups of the population with differing exercise levels provide sufficient evidence to advocate regular moderate physical exercise throughout life (see Chapters 5 and 11)*.

Accidents

Accidents are a major cause of death and disability. There are clear differences in the risk of accidents related to age and social class. In particular, accidents take a tragic toll in young children, in whom they

---

*See also *Exercise: benefits and risks*. A report of a working party of the Royal College of Physicians 1991.

are the commonest cause of death, and in the elderly. Accidents in teenagers and young adults, often related to risk-taking and consumption of alcohol, are also an important cause of death and injury.

The effects of various control measures by education, by environmental change and by enforcement are hard to measure, although the role of some specific actions such as seat belt legislation, can be fairly accurately assessed. Nevertheless, the reduction in death rates from accidents does suggest that preventive measures have an effect.

Problems requiring further efforts at prevention include: pedestrian road traffic accidents, burns and scalds in children, car occupant and motor cycle accidents in teenagers and young adults, accidents at work and in leisure activities, and all forms of home accidents especially in the elderly.

Some scope for advance lies in environmental improvements, for example in road speeds, and with legislative action, but the most important factor in reducing accidents is likely to be changes in attitudes and behaviour in relation to known causes of accidents such as drink driving.

Health staff have an important educational role in providing useful and accurate information, by screening for conditions such as alcoholism which contribute to risk of accidents, and by training in first aid and resuscitation.

Occupational disease

The impact of occupational ill-health is imperfectly measured and difficult to assess. Although the classical occupational diseases such as cancers related to industrial exposure are well recognised, there is evidence of substantial under-reporting even of these well-defined conditions. In addition, there is an ill-defined but certainly large burden of ill-health related to occupation but not specific to it. Musculo-skeletal and psychiatric disorders are especially relevant here, but many skin, respiratory, vascular and neurological disorders, and some cancers (other than those ordinarily recognised as occupational) may have an occupational element in their causation.

The present methods of control comprise a mixture of risk assessment, control and monitoring within industry, pre-employment screening to exclude workers who have health problems putting them at increased risk, and health promotion for employees, together with a strong legislative framework. This combination of measures has been notably successful but there is a need for continued research as industrial and employment practices change. Further efforts are needed also to improve information available about occupational ill-health and to evaluate control measures. There is much scope for improved education on occupational risk, both for the public and the medical profession.

Measures to protect against the carcinogenic effects of excess ultra-violet and ionising radiation are important both for specific occupations and for the public generally.

Screening

Although many diagnostic tests are available to test apparently well people for unsuspected disease, caution needs to be applied in recommending widespread screening. It cannot be assumed that because a disease is detected before symptoms occur, the prognosis following treatment is necessarily improved. Some of the screen-detected cases may already be incurable while some others would have been curable even if not diagnosed until later when symptoms had arisen. More than other preventive measures, screening is likely to harm some of the well people tested, especially those with borderline or false positive results, and some people with early disease will not be detected because their test result is a false negative. For these reasons screening needs to be tested on a trial basis for each disease and each screening test to find out what proportion of morbidity and mortality it can prevent and at what price in terms of causing morbidity as well as using resources. Unfortunately, in the past this requirement to evaluate was often neglected and many established screening programmes are of uncertain benefit and unknown cost, indicating the need for further research. Many of the abnormalities for which screening may be advocated are not early manifestations of disease so much as risk indicators of later disease: eg hypertension as a risk factor for stroke, plasma cholesterol as a risk factor for coronary heart disease. These risk factor tests tend to have both poor specificity (many false positives) and poor sensitivity (many false negatives) when judged against the gold-standard of incidence of future disease. It is therefore imperative that their cost-effectiveness should be established by adequately designed randomised controlled trials.

Screening during pregnancy Screening tests to detect various fetal abnormalities (eg neural tube defects and Down's syndrome) and inherited disorders (eg Duchenne muscular dystrophy and cystic fibrosis), followed by termination, if requested, of pregnancies with an affected fetus, can reduce the prevalence of these disorders. This subject has not been reviewed in depth in this report*. Screening for

*For fuller review see: *Prenatal diagnosis and genetic screening: community and service implications*. A report of a working party of the Royal College of Physicians 1989.

maternal infections such as syphilis and hepatitis B in order to treat the mother and prevent infection of the fetus or infant is recommended. But the benefit of routine screening for toxoplasmosis and cytomegalovirus infection is questionable. Screening for maternal rubella infection, with the option of termination of pregnancy for those found to have had an active infection during the first trimester, is advisable for women who have been exposed to the infection, and selective HIV screening for women at risk must also now be considered.

Neonatal screening Screening for phenylketonuria and for congenital hypothyroidism with subsequent maintenance treatment for cases identified, are effective in prevention of mental handicap. Screening for congenital dislocation of the hip is of uncertain benefit. Detection of other congenital abnormalities before they cause symptoms, eg structural heart abnormalities, may be beneficial but has not been fully evaluated.

Screening in infancy and childhood Screening for hearing loss is accepted as being beneficial, particularly in infancy when appropriate sound amplification may enable normal speech development. Detection of 'glue ear' is of uncertain benefit because the condition tends to resolve spontaneously, and treatment by myringotomy with grommets may cause long-term damage. Visual screening, for amblyopia in early childhood, and in school children for myopia and in boys colour blindness, is accepted as beneficial. Research into the effectiveness of general surveillance of growth and development of children is a high priority.

Pre-employment medical examinations The purpose of these is to determine whether the person is fit for the occupational task rather than to alter long-term prognosis by early detection of asymptomatic disease. Similarly, monitoring of various physical attributes during the course of employment (eg hearing levels for those in noisy jobs) is done so that the person with signs of early disease may be moved away from the exposure to prevent further deterioration, rather than to instigate early treatment.

Smoking and alcohol history These are screening tests for risk factors for many diseases. They have not been formally evaluated in terms of their effectiveness in reducing morbidity and mortality. Nevertheless, history-taking is an entirely safe and very cheap method of identifying people at risk. Moreover, experimental evidence that casefinding and subsequent advice achieves long-term cessation in a proportion of cases, at least for cigarette smoking, makes such history-taking a recommended practice for reducing the toll of tobacco and alcohol-related disease.

Screening for hypertension   Randomised controlled trials have demonstrated that drug treatment of asymptomatic hypertension is effective
in reducing subsequent incidence of stroke (but not coronary heart
disease). Case-finding of asymptomatic hypertension in primary care
settings is therefore recommended, with routine blood-pressure measurements at 5-yearly intervals. However, because hypertension is only a
risk factor, rather than an early manifestation of stroke, the cost-
effectiveness of this screening is debatable. Non-pharmacological control
of mild hypertension should always be tried before putting a patient
on antihypertensive drugs. A priority area for further research is the
cost-effectiveness of hypertension screening in later life.

Screening for plasma cholesterol level   In asymptomatic patients with high
cholesterol levels treatment with cholesterol lowering drugs has been
shown to be effective in reducing subsequent coronary heart disease.
Screening and early treatment of people with less extreme levels of
raised plasma cholesterol is more controversial because of the poor
sensitivity and specificity of this test in predicting future coronary heart
disease, when it is not accompanied by other coronary risk factors,
because of the lack of resources for dietary counselling of those with
positive results, and because of the costs of life-long drug treatment.
Cholesterol screening by case-finding within primary care settings for
patients with a history of familial hyper-cholesterolaemia, and those
with already recognised further risk factors for coronary heart disease
(eg smoking habit, hypertension, exercise habit) is recommended. But
no system for monitoring the implementation of this policy (eg the
criteria used by different doctors for estimating whether a person is or
is not at risk), nor for evaluating its cost-effectiveness yet exists.

Screening for prevention of cervical cancer   Cytological examination of
cervical smears can identify cervical intra-epithelial neoplasia (CIN)
which is an indicator of very high risk of invasive cancer. The evidence
suggests that detection and elimination of CIN 3 in a 3–5-yearly
screening programme could prevent 90% of invasive cancers up to age
65. Such a level of effectiveness has not been achieved in the UK mainly
because of poor coverage of women above the reproductive age-group.
The cost-effectiveness of ablative treatment of lesser degrees of CIN is
unknown. Screening is recommended at 3- to 5-yearly intervals for all
women aged 20 to 64 years, and for older women who have not had two
negative cervical smear results in the previous decade. Screening more
often than 3-yearly is not cost-effective.

Screening for breast cancer   Randomised controlled trials have shown that
20% to 30% of deaths from breast cancer between the ages of about 55

and 74 years could be avoided by screening. The current UK screening programme provides 3-yearly screening for all women aged 50 to 64, who should be encouraged to participate in it. Screening younger women, and screening more frequently, are the subjects of current research projects.

Screening for other cancers   Screening for lung cancer has been shown to be ineffective in several trials. Screening for testicular cancer is probably unnecessary because the cure rate for symptomatic disease is now so good. Screening for numerous other sites of cancer (large bowel, stomach, ovary, bladder, melanoma of the skin, prostate, neuroblastoma) is still of unproven benefit.

Screening for unreported disabilities in the elderly   While much can be done by anticipatory care of elderly patients (eg anticoagulant treatment of those with atrial fibrillation) the benefits and hazards of formal screening programmes still need to be evaluated (see Chapter 11).

Childhood

The health of children in Britain has improved greatly during this century, with a dramatic and continued reduction in perinatal, infant and childhood mortality. Much of this change is associated with social, environmental and nutritional improvements not directly related to medical interventions but some, notably immunisation, are of proven benefit. There is also clear evidence that modern obstetric practice and technical care of the new born has led to improving perinatal mortality and morbidity. Nevertheless, many illnesses causing death and disability remain uncontrolled, some such as diabetes and asthma, appear to be increasing, and the survival of children with previously fatal conditions has increased the prevalence of some forms of chronic disability.

The effects of social and environmental disadvantage, detectable in many aspects of health at all ages, are especially important in infancy and childhood. The associations between disadvantage and health are related to markers such as extremes of maternal age, poor parental education, high birth order and lack of support for mothers, and are often also associated with poor housing and other stressful life circumstances. The associated childhood health problems include an undue burden of respiratory and other infections, accidents and developmental and behavioural problems. Social class-related differences in infant mortality have remained unchanged since 1950.

Of the medical preventive activities applicable in childhood, many are of proven benefit and others, while less firmly established as effective, are certainly worth promoting on the available evidence. Table 10.1 lists these two categories of intervention, showing especially the value of the immunisation programme and of certain forms of screening and dietary interventions, and the likely benefits of a number of other preventive actions. What is now needed is increased recognition of the likely benefits to the health of children and their future adult lives if the measures known to be beneficial are rigorously implemented and further knowledge gained. Among those needing special attention are:

- improved integration of child health services
- improved information systems on child health
- promotion of immunisation programmes
- evaluation of screening programmes
- further work on content and delivery of educational programmes aimed at health education for children, parents and health care workers
- special attention to education and delivery of health care to children with special needs and those from deprived backgrounds.

Later life

The aim of preventive medicine in old age is to prevent disability. It is to be hoped—and there is some evidence to support this—that if health can be preserved and disability can be prevented into old age, the period of ultimate dependency may be shortened. A sad exception is found in the increasing survival time of patients with dementia.

It has often been assumed that preventive measures aimed at external factors thought to be cumulative in their effects, for example, cholesterol levels, will have no role in the elderly, but there is some evidence that interventions of this sort may also be effective in old age. It is certainly reasonable for elderly people to stop smoking and to adopt sensible diets.

It is likely that maintaining active mental and physical activities and social contacts is conducive to the prevention of disability in old age. The role of physical exercise is likely to be important, by reducing bone loss, maintaining muscle function, and diminishing joint stiffness. All these effects, together with hormone replacement therapy in post-menopausal women, will help to reduce the risk of falls and fractures.

Of the specifically medical preventive actions, the role of drugs in causing, as well as relieving problems in the elderly, needs special attention, as also does the role of anticoagulant therapy in atrial fibrillation and the role of vitamin D.

Many aspects of prevention in old age need further study. These include especially the effect of interventions which are of established value in younger age groups, the ill-effects of cold and nutritional problems in the elderly short of obvious malnutrition.

Health education related to the elderly should be aimed, not only at the elderly, but at younger age groups and the health professions, in order to counteract dismissive attitudes to disability in the elderly, and to show the positive aspects of prevention in the older age groups. Elderly people should be encouraged to expect and require high standards of health care.

Economic aspects of curtailing consumption of alcohol and tobacco

The tenor of this report is that there are great potential benefits to be achieved from reduced consumption of alcohol and tobacco. These are largely in the form of health gains, but several important economic benefits such as reduced health care costs and increased industrial output due to less sickness absence from work were also cited.

While it would be wrong to imply that reductions in cigarette and alcohol consumption might not also impose economic costs, some of the economic arguments which have been used in support of smoking and drinking are spurious. This appendix examines four attributes of tobacco and alcohol which have been used to defend smoking and drinking on economic grounds. These are:

1. Both are major sources of government revenue;
2. Both employ thousands of people directly in the production of tobacco and alcohol products and indirectly through retail sales, advertising etc;
3. As a cause of premature death they restrict the number of elderly people in the population who consume a disproportionate amount of health and social services and who have to be supported by pensions;
4. Tobacco exports are a major source of income to many developing countries.

These are discussed here in turn.

Government revenue

There are two principal reasons why government taxes alcohol and tobacco: as a means of collecting revenue and as a means of controlling consumption.

Economic studies indicate that the demand for tobacco and alcohol are 'inelastic' (a rise in price causes a smaller proportionate fall in consumption). This means that raising duty will have the effect of both reducing consumption and, at the same time, raising government revenue. The public health and revenue raising roles of government are here mutually supportive.

Despite this, there are several reasons why government may not wish to increase these duties. First, it can be argued that further increases would be 'unfair'. Smokers and drinkers currently pay more in duties than the extra costs of health care and lost output due to smoking/drinking related illness which they impose. Second, these duties are 'regressive' taxes in that they are not related to ability to pay and therefore hurt the poor more than the rich. Additionally, recent evidence suggests that increases in tobacco duty induce greater falls in consumption by the higher social classes than the lower. Government has the ability to collect revenue in more 'progressive' ways, eg by raising income taxes. Third, tobacco and alcohol are both items included in the Retail Price Index. Raising duties is therefore inflationary.

While a reduction in smoking and drinking which results from increased taxation will raise government revenue, a reduction for any other reason, eg health education, will cause government revenue to fall. Here the public health role of government is in potential conflict with its revenue raising role.

The Treasury currently earns £6,000 million per year from tobacco duty and £7,300 million per year from alcohol duties. Together, these represent more than half the total cost of the National Health Service. From the point of view of the economy, these sums should not be regarded as either good or bad things. Tobacco and alcohol duties are what are referred to as 'transfer payments'. They are not related to the resource cost of producing the products, but are merely ways of transferring cash from one pocket to another. They are, of course, 'costs' to the smoker and drinker who pays them, but they generate identical 'benefits' to the government which collects them. If people suddenly and completely stopped smoking and drinking, then government would have some £13,300 million less to spend on schools, roads and health care, but (ex)smokers and more moderate drinkers would have £13,300 million more to spend in other ways. (Note that this is independent of the money which the tobacco and alcohol companies receive in return for producing the products). The economy as a whole would be worse off only to the extent that some of this extra money in the hands of consumers may be saved or spent on imports.

The impact on government revenue of reduced smoking and drinking is likely to be less severe than may be imagined. If these sources of revenue were suddenly stopped, government would indeed be in difficult circumstances. Other forms of revenue would have to be found quickly or there would have to be major cutbacks in government expenditure. However, a sudden ending of tobacco revenue or a dramatic decline in alcohol revenue is most unlikely even under the most optimistic assumptions of the success of anti-smoking and moderate drinking programmes. A gradual reduction, which is more likely, would give government time to adjust other taxes to make up for the fall in revenue.

Employment

Unlike tobacco and alcohol duties, jobs in the tobacco and alcohol industries (strictly it is the value of the output produced) and the related areas they support, are true economic benefits to the nation. Loss of jobs due to reduced smoking and drinking represents true costs, although, unless unemployment is high, these freed labour resources could be put to other productive uses. Furthermore, as future falls in the demand for cigarettes and alcohol are likely to be relatively gradual, output reductions are also likely to be gradual. Much of the money not spent on these products will be spent elsewhere, thus increasing the demand for other goods and the demand for labour to produce them.

The 'benefit' of early death

As most elderly people are no longer economically productive, it might be argued that they impose a burden on the economy by receiving pensions and consuming disproportionate amounts of health and social services. It may therefore appear that somehow the life years gained by reduced smoking and moderate drinking should be regarded as dis-benefits.

As stated in the introduction to this Report, prevention may save resources, but this is not its primary objective. As with treatment, prevention can be efficient without saving money. Society does not value human life solely for its economic productivity. This is clear from the large amounts of resources willingly spent on those members of society who are not economically active, the unemployable for example, or those mentally or physically disabled people who in economic terms will inevitably consume more than they produce. Years of life gained from reductions in smoking or drinking must therefore be regarded as benefits. Moreover, the age of retirement and its associated unproduct-ivity is arbitrarily imposed and could conceivably be changed.

The economy of developing nations

Though it cannot be denied that tobacco represents a major source of income to many countries, the resources currently devoted to raising tobacco could be used for the cultivation of other crops. Indeed it can equally be argued that a shift toward the production of other food crops could, in the long run, be more beneficial to the countries involved.

Balance of gains and losses

Against these real and perceived economic costs of reduced smoking and drinking have to be considered the economic gains which include: reducing the £500 million currently spent on treating smoking related diseases and the £150 million per year spent on treating alcohol related disease, reducing the current £700 million burden to industry of sickness absence due to smoking and £1,000 million per year due to alcohol, plus many additional avoidable costs such as fires caused by cigarettes and the crime and other social problems resulting from alcohol misuse.

While reduced smoking and drinking will have some negative economic aspects, the overall economic consequence will be favourable. Given the enormous health gains potentially achievable, the economic effects add support to the call for further legislative action as well as an increase in health education and clinical preventive activity.

References

Chapter 2: **Smoking**

1. Corti, Count EC (1931) *A history of smoking.* London: Harrap.
2. Office of Population Censuses and Surveys (1990). *Cigarette smoking 1972 to 1988.* OPCS Monitor SS90/2. London: HMSO.
3. Doll R, Hill AB (1950) Smoking and carcinoma of the lung. *British Medical Journal,* **ii**, 739.
4. Wynder EL, Graham EA (1950) Tobacco smoking as a possible aetiological factor in bronchogenic carcinoma. *Journal of the American Medical Association,* **143**, 329.
5. Doll R, Peto R (1976) Mortality in relation to smoking: 20 years' observation on British male doctors. *British Medical Journal,* **iv**, 1525.
6. Doll R, Gray R, Hafner B, Peto R (1980) Mortality in relation to smoking: 22 years' observation on female British doctors. *British Medical Journal,* **i**, 967.
7. Hammond EC (1966) Smoking in relation to the death rates of one million men and women. In: National Cancer Institute Monograph (ed. W Haenzel), **19**, 127.
8. Hammond EC, Horn D (1958) Smoking and death rates: Report of 44 months of follow-up of 187,783 men. *Journal of the American Medical Association,* **166**, 1159, 1294.
9. Royal College of Physicians (1962) *Smoking and health.* London: Pitman Medical.
10. Royal College of Physicians (1983) *Smoking or health?* London: Pitman.
11. Peto R (1980) Possible ways of explaining to ordinary people the quantitative dangers of smoking. *Health Education Journal,* **39**, 45.
12. Froggatt P (1988) *Fourth report of Independent Scientific Committee on Smoking and Health.* London: HMSO.
13. Colley JRT (1974) Respiratory symptoms in children and parental smoking and phlegm production. *British Medical Journal,* **ii**, 201.
14. White JR, Froeb H (1980) Small airways dysfunction in non-smokers chronically exposed to tobacco smoke. *New England Journal of Medicine,* **302**, 720.
15. Wald NJ, Nanchatal K, Cuckle H (1983) Does breathing other people's smoke cause lung cancer? *British Medical Journal,* **293**, 1217.
16. Ashton H, Stepney R (1982) *Smoking: psychology and pharmacology.* London: Tavistock Publications.
17. Marsh A, Matheson J (1983) *Smoking attitudes and behaviour.* London: HMSO.
18. Fowler G, Mant D, Fuller A, Jones L (1989) The 'Help Your Patient Stop' initiative. *Lancet,* **i**, 1253.
19. Wallace PG, Haines AP (1984) General practitioners and health promotion: What patients think. *British Medical Journal,* **289**, 354.
20. McCron R, Budd J (1979) *Communication and health education.* Unpublished document prepared for Health Education Council. Leicester: University of Leicester Centre for Mass Communication Research.

21. Russell MAH, Wilson C, Taylor C, Baker CD (1979) Effect of general practitioners' advice against smoking. *British Medical Journal*, **2**, 231.
22. Jamrozik K, Vessey M, Fowler G *et al.* (1984) Controlled trial of three different anti-smoking interventions in general practice. *British Medical Journal*, **288**, 1499.
23. Richmond R, Austin A, Webster I (1986) Three year evaluation of a programme by general practitioners to help patients stop smoking. *British Medical Journal*, **292**, 803.
24. Williams A (1987) Screening for risk of CHD: is it wise use of resources? In *Screening for risk of coronary heart disease* (eds M Oliver, M Ashley-Miller, D Wood). Chichester: Wiley.
25. Cummings SR, Rubin SM, Oster G (1989) The cost-effectiveness of counselling smokers to quit. *Journal of the American Medical Association*, **261**, 75.
26. Raw M (1985) Does nicotine chewing gum work? *British Medical Journal*, **290**, 1231.
27. Chapman S (1985) Stop-smoking clinics: a case for their abandonment. *Lancet*, **i**, 918.
28. Kunze M, Wood M (eds) (1984) *Guidelines on smoking cessation*. Geneva: UICC.
29. Goddard E (1989) *Smoking among secondary school children in England in 1988*. London: HMSO.

Further reading

Help your patient stop: this booklet, published by the British Medical Association and Imperial Cancer Fund (and available from the BMA), is a useful, simple guide on smoking cessation for primary health care teams.

Chapter 3: **Alcohol**

1. Taylor D (1981) *Alcohol: reducing the harm*. London: Office of Health Economics.
2. McDonnell R, Maynard A (1985) The costs of alcohol misuse. *British Journal of Addiction*, **80**, 27.
3. Royal College of Physicians (1987) *The medical consequences of alcohol abuse: a great and growing evil*. A report of a working party. London: Tavistock Publications.
4. Royal College of Psychiatrists (1986) *Alcohol – our favourite drug*. Report of a Special Committee. London: Tavistock Publications.
5. Royal College of General Practitioners (1986) *Alcohol, a balanced view*. London: Royal College of General Practitioners.
6. British Medical Association (1988) *ABC of alcohol* (ed. A Paton) London: British Medical Journal.
7. Faculty of Public Health Medicine (1991) *Alcohol and the public health*. London: Macmillan.
8. Orford J, Harwin J (eds) (1982) *Alcohol and the family*. London: Croom Helm.
9. Hore BD, Plant MA (eds) (1981) *Alcohol problems in employment*. London: Croom Helm.

10. Sabey BE, Staughton GC (1980) *The drinking road user in Great Britain.* Crowthorne, Berks: Transport and Road Research Laboratory.
11. Greenberg SW (1982) Alcohol and crime: A methodological critique of the literature. In: *Drinking and crime: perspectives on the relationship between alcohol consumption and criminal behaviour* (ed. JJ Colins). London: Tavistock Publications.
12. Office of Population Censuses and Surveys (1986) *Occupational mortality, decennial supplement,* No 6, 1979–80, 1982–83. London: HMSO.
13. Papoz L, Weill J, L'Hoste J, *et al.* (1986) Biological markers of alcohol intake among 4796 subjects injured in accidents. *British Medical Journal,* **292**, 1234.
14. Rada RT (1975) Alcoholism and rape. *American Journal of Psychiatry,* **132**, 444.
15. Riley D (1984) Drivers' beliefs about alcohol and the law. *Home Office Research Bulletin,* No 17. London: Home Office.
16. British Medical Association (1986) *Young people and alcohol.* Report of the Board of Science and Education of the BMA. London: Chameleon Press.
17. Jackson R, Scragg R, Beaglehole R (1991) Alcohol consumption and risk of coronary heart disease. *British Medical Journal,* **303**, 211.
18. Ledermann S (1956) *Alcool, alcoolism et alcoolisation.* Paris: Vol Press Universitaires de France.
19. Popham RE, Schmidt W, de Lint L (1975) The prevention of alcoholism: epidemiological studies of the effect of government control measures. *British Journal of Addiction,* **70**, 125.
20. Jones B, Jones M (1976) Intoxication, metabolism and the menstrual cycle. In: *Alcoholism problems in women and children* (eds Greenblatt and Shukitt). New York: Grune and Stratton.
21. Frezza M, Di Padova C, Pozzato G *et al.* (1990) High blood alcohol levels in women. *New England Journal of Medicine,* **322**, 95.
22. Wilkinson P, Kornaczewski A, Rankin JG, Santa Maria JN (1971) Physical disease and alcoholism: initial survey of 1,000 population. *Medical Journal of Australia,* **1**, 1217.
23. Williams R, Davis M (1977) Alcoholic liver diseases – basic pathology and clinical variants. In: *Alcoholism: new knowledge and new responses* (eds G Edwards and M Grant). London: Croom Helm.
24. Cust G (1980) Health education about alcohol in the Tyne Tees area. In: *Aspects of alcohol and drug dependence* (eds TS Madden *et al.*). Tunbridge Wells: Pitman Medical.
25. Nielson DD, Sorensen DD (1979) Alcohol policy: alcohol consumption, alcohol prices, delirium tremens and alcoholism as cause of death in Denmark. *Social Psychiatry,* **14**, 133.

Chapter 4: **Healthy diets**

1. Doll R (1989) The prevalence of cancer: opportunities and challenges. In *Reducing the risk of cancer* (eds T Heller, B Davey, L Bailey). London: Hodder and Stoughton.
2. Office of Population Censuses and Surveys (1988) *Mortality statistics: cause. England and Wales 1988,* Series DH2 No. 16. London: HMSO.

3. NACNE (1983) *A discussion paper on proposals for nutritional guidelines for health education in Britain.* London: Health Education Council.
4. Bender AE, Brookes LJ (eds) (1987). *Body weight control.* Proceedings of the First International Meeting on Body Weight Control, Montreux, Switzerland, April 1985. London: Churchill Livingstone.
5. Garrow JS (1988) *Obesity and related diseases.* London: Churchill Livingstone.
6. Committee of Medical Aspects of Food Policy (1991) *Dietary reference values for food energy and nutrients for the UK.* London: HMSO.
7. Garrow JS (1991) Nutrition. In *Oxford textbook of public health*, 2nd edn (eds WW Holland, R Detels, EG Knox), Vol 1, Ch 6 (Influences of public health). Oxford: Oxford University Press.
8. Knight I (1989) The heights and weights of adults in Great Britain, 1984. *Social Trends*, **19**.
9. Adams CE, Morgan KJ (1981) Periodicity of eating: implications for human food consumption. *Nutrition Research*, **1**, 525.
10. James WPT (1988) *Health nutrition: preventing nutrition-related diseases in Europe.* World Health Organisation Regional Publications, European series, No. 24. Copenhagen: WHO Regional Office for Europe.
11. Committee on Medical Aspects of Food Policy (1984) *Diet and cardiovascular disease.* Report on health and social subjects, No. 28. Department of Health and Social Security. London: HMSO.
12. Mann JL *et al.* (1988) Blood lipid concentration and other cardiovascular risk factor distribution, prevalence and detection in Britain. *British Medical Journal*, **396**, 1702.
13. Office of Medical Applications of Research, National Institutes of Health (1985) Lowering blood cholesterol to prevent heart disease. *Journal of the American Medical Association*, **253**, 2080.
14. Gurr ML *et al.* (1989) Dietary fat and plasma lipids. *Nutrition Research Reviews*, **2**, 63.
15. Morris JN *et al.* (1977) Diet and heart – a postscript. *British Medical Journal*, **2**, 1307.
16. Kushi LH *et al.* (1985) Diet and 20 year mortality from CHD. The Ireland-Boston diet heart study. *New England Journal of Medicine*, **312** (13), 811.
17. World Health Organisation (1982) *Prevention of coronary heart disease: report of a WHO Expert Committee.* WHO Technical Report series No. 678. Geneva: WHO.
18. Intersalt Cooperative Research Group (1988) Intersalt: an international study of electrolyte excretion and blood pressure. Results for 24-hour sodium and potassium excretion. *British Medical Journal*, **297**, 319.
19. Law MR, Frost CD, Wald NJ (1991) By how much does dietary salt reduction lower blood pressure? *British Medical Journal*, **302**, 811.
20. Heaton KW (1990) Dietary fibre. *British Medical Journal*, **200**, 1480.
21. Ministry of Agriculture Fisheries and Food (1985) *Manual of nutrition.* London: HMSO.
22. Truswell AS (1986) In: *ABC of nutrition.* London: BMJ.
23. MRC Vitamin Study Research Group (1991) Prevention of neural tube defects: results of the Medical Research Council Vitamin Study. *Lancet*, **338**, 131.
24. Royal College of Physicians of London (1976) *Fluoride, teeth and health*, Report of a working party. London: Pitman Medical.

25. Department of Health and Social Security (1979) *Eating for health*. London: DHSS.
26. Royal College of Physicians of London (1984) *Food intolerance and food aversion*. Report of a Working Party. London: Royal College of Physicians.
27. Royal College of Physicians of London (1987) *Medical aspects of food intolerance*. A group of papers based on a survey. London: Royal College of Physicians.
28. Department of Health and Social Security Advisory Committee on Irradiated and Novel Foods (1986) *Report on the safety and wholesomeness of irradiation of food*. London: HMSO.
29. Central Statistical Office (1989) Fatty acid content of the average British diet. *Social Trends*, **19**, 122. London: HMSO.
30. Central Statistical Office (1989) *Social Trends*, **19**. London: HMSO.

Chapter 5: **Heart disease and stroke**

1. Office of Population Censuses and Surveys (1990) *Deaths by cause: 1989 registrations*. London: OPCS.
2. Maynard A, Hardman G, Godfrey C (1989) *Priorities for health promotion: an economic appraisal*. Discussion paper 55. Centre for Health Economics, University of York.
3. Pekkanen J, Linn S, Heiss G *et al.* (1990) Ten-year mortality from cardiovascular disease in relation to cholesterol level among men with and without pre-existing cardiovascular disease. *New England Journal of Medicine*, **322**, 1700.
4. Royal College of Physicians (1976) Smoking. In: Joint working party report *Prevention of coronary heart disease*, p 20. London: Royal College of Physicians.
5. Meade TW, North WRS, Chakrabartir *et al.* (1980) Haemostatic function and cardiovascular death: early results of a prospective study. *Lancet*, **i**, 1050.
6. Paffenbarger RS, Wing AL, Hyde RT (1978) Physical activity as an index of heart attack risk in college alumni. *American Journal of Epidemiology*, **108**, 161.
7. Royal College of Physicians (1991) *Medical aspects of exercise – benefits and risks*. Report of a working party. London: Royal College of Physicians.
8. Yusuf S, Cutler J (1987) Single factor trials drug studies. In *Atherosclerosis: biology and clinical science* (ed. AG Olsson), p 393. Edinburgh: Churchill Livingstone.
9. British Cardiac Society (1987) *Report of British Cardiac Society working group on coronary disease prevention*. London: British Cardiac Society.
10. European Atherosclerosis Society (1987) Strategies for the prevention of coronary heart disease. *European Heart Journal*, **8**, 77.
11. The Steering Committee of the Physicians Health Study Research Group (1989) Final report on the aspirin component of the ongoing Physicians' Health Study. *New England Journal of Medicine*, **321**, 129.
12. Thom TJ (1989) International mortality from heart disease: rates and trends. *International Journal of Epidemiology*, **18** (suppl 1), 520.
13. MacMahon S, Peto R, Cutler J *et al.* (1990) Blood pressure and coronary heart disease. Part 1. Prolonged differences in blood pressure: prospective

observation studies corrected for the regression dilution bias. *Lancet*, **335**, 765.

14. Collins R, Peto R, MacMahon S *et al* (1990) Blood pressure, stroke and coronary heart disease. Part 2. Short-term reductions in blood pressure: overview of randomised trials in their epidemiological context. *Lancet*, **335**, 827.

15. Medical Research Council working party (1985) MRC trial of treatment of mild hypertension. *British Medical Journal*, **291**, 97.

16. World Health Organisation (1989) Guidelines for the management of mild hypertension: memorandum from a WHO/ISM meeting. *Bulletin of the World Health Organisation*, **67**, 493.

Chapter 6: **Cancer**

1. Doll R, Peto R (1981) *The causes of cancer*. Oxford: Oxford University Press.

2. Davis DL, Hoel D, Fox J, Lopez A (1990) International trends in cancer mortality in France, West Germany, Italy, Japan, England and Wales and the USA. *Lancet*, **2**, 474.

3. Peto R (1989) The future effects caused by smoking. In: *Tobacco or health: the way ahead*. Proceedings of the first European Conference on Tobacco Policy. Copenhagen: WHO Regional Office for Europe.

4. Miller AB (ed) (1989) *Diet and the aetiology of cancer*. European School of Oncology Monographs.

5. Doll R (1989) The prevention of cancer: opportunities and challenges. In: *Reducing the risk of cancers* (eds T Heller *et al.*). London: Hodder & Stoughton.

6. Mackie R, Elwood JM, Hawk JLM (1987) Links between exposure to ultraviolet radiation and skin cancer. A report. *Journal of the Royal College of Physicians of London*, **21**, 91.

7. International Agency for Research on Cancer (1987) *Evaluation of carcinogenic risks to humans*. IARC monographs, Suppl 7. Lyon: IARC.

8. Commins BT (1989) Estimations of risk from environmental asbestos in perspective. In *Non-occupational exposure to mineral fibres*. IARC Scientific Publication, No. 90, p 476. Lyon: IARC.

9. Day NE (1989) Screening for cancer of the cervix. *Journal of Epidemiology and Community Health*, **43**, 103.

10. Ellman R, Chamberlain J (1984) Improving the effectiveness of cervical cancer screening. *Journal of the Royal College of General Practitioners*, **34**, 537.

11. Shapiro S, Venet W, Strax P, Venet L (1988) *Periodic screening for breast cancer: The Health Insurance Plan Project and its sequelae, 1963–1986*. Baltimore: Johns Hopkins University Press.

12. Tabar L, Fagemberg G, Duffy SW, Day NE (1989) The Swedish two-county trial of mammographic screening for breast cancer: recent results and calculations of benefit. *Journal of Epidemiology and Community Health*, **43**, 107.

13. Forrest APM (1990) *The decision to screen*. London: Nuffield Provincial Hospitals Trust.

14. Early Detection of Breast Cancer Group (1988) First results on mortality reduction in the UK trial of early detection of breast cancer. *Lancet*, **2**, 411.

15. Ellman R, Angeli N, Christians A *et al.* (1989) Psychiatric morbidity associated with screening for breast cancer. *British Journal of Cancer*, **60**, 781.
16. Brett GZ (1968) The value of lung cancer detection by six-monthly chest radiographs. *Thorax*, **23**, 414.
17. Fontana RS, Sanderson DR, Woolner LB *et al.* (1986) Lung cancer screening: the Mayo program. *Journal of Occupational Medicine*, **28**, 746.
18. Kubik A, Parkin DM, Khlat M *et al.* (1990) Lack of benefit from semi-annual screening for cancer of the lung. *International Journal of Cancer*, **45**, 26.

Chapter 7: **Infectious disease**

1. Brown F (1990) From Jenner to genes – the new vaccines. *Lancet*, **335**, 587.
2. Noah ND (1982) Measles eradication policies. *British Medical Journal*, **284**, 997.
3. Department of Health (1990) *Immunisation against infectious disease*. London: HMSO.
4. Ferguson M (1990) Hepatitis vaccines. *Current Opinion in Infectious Diseases*, **3**, 367.
5. Noah ND (1988) Vaccination against pneumococcal infection. *British Medical Journal*, **297**, 1351.
6. Elliman D (1989) Adverse reactions and immunization schedules. *Current Opinion in Infectious Diseases*, **2**, 773.
7. Robbins A (1990) Progress towards vaccines we need and do not have. *Lancet*, **335**, 1436.
8. Polakoff S (1983) The use of immunoglobulins in virus infections. In *Recent advances in clinical virology* (ed AP Waterson), Ch 6. Edinburgh: Churchill Livingstone.
9. Pollock AV (1988) Surgical prophylaxis: the emerging picture. In *Infection today*. A *Lancet* review, p 99.
10. Meers P, Ayliffe GA, Emmerson AM *et al* (1981) Report of the National Survey of Infection in Hospitals – 1980. *Journal of Hospital Infection* (supplement).
11. Finch R (1988) Minimising the risk of legionnaires' disease. *British Medical Journal*, **296**, 1343.
12. Behrens RH (1990) Protecting the health of the international traveller. *Transactions of the Royal Society of Tropical Medicine and Hygiene*, **84**, 611, 629.
13. Roberts D (1990) Sources of infection: food. *Lancet*, **336**, 859.
14. Gill ON, Bartlett CLR, Sockett PN *et al* (1983) Outbreak of *Salmonella napoli* infection caused by contaminated chocolate bars. *Lancet*, **i**, 574.
15. Rowe B, Begg NT, Hutchinson DN *et al* (1987) Salmonella ealing infections associated with consumption of infant dried milk. *Lancet*, **ii**, 900.
16. Richmond Committee (1990) *The microbiological safety of food*, Part 1. London: HMSO.
17. Collee JG (1990) Bovine spongiform encephalopathy. *Lancet*, **336**, 1300.
18. WJ Eylenbosch, ND Noah (eds) (1988) In *Surveillance in health and disease*, Ch 2. Oxford: Oxford University Press.

Further reading

Before you go. The traveller's guide to health, SA 40. *While you're away. The traveller's guide to health*, SA 41. (Two pamphlets prepared by the Department of Health and the Central Office of Information. Published by HMSO.)

Health information for international travel 1990. Centers for disease control. US Department of Health and Human Services.

Chapter 8: **Accidents**

1. Royal College of Surgeons of England (1989) *Accident prevention: a social responsibility*. London: Royal College of Surgeons.
2. Office of Population Censuses and Surveys. *Deaths from accidents and violence*. London: OPCS Monitor Series DH4 (Published quarterly).
3. Royal College of Physicians (1989) *Fractured neck of femur: prevention and management*. Report of a Working Party. London: Royal College of Physicians.
4. Automobile Association Foundation for Road Safety Research (1989) *Motoring and the older driver*. Basingstoke: AA.
5. Department of Transport (1991) *Road accidents in Great Britain 1990. The casualty report*. London: HMSO.
6. Child Accident Prevention Trust (1989) *Basic principles of child accident prevention. A guide to action*. London: Child Accident Prevention Trust.
7. Department of Transport (1990) *Children and roads: a safer way*. London: Department of Transport.
8. National Association of Health Authorities/Royal Society for the Prevention of Accidents (1990) *The role of health authorities in accident prevention*. Birmingham: National Association of Health Authorities.
9. British Medical Association/The Pharmaceutical Society of Great Britain. *British National Formulary* (Published annually).
10. Medical Commission on Accident Prevention (1985) *Medical aspects of fitness to drive* (4th edn). London: Medical Commission on Accident Prevention.

Chapter 9: **Occupational medicine**

1. Ramazzini B (1713) *De Morbis Artificum* (2nd edn) (Translated by WC Wright 1940). Chicago: Chicago University Press.
2. Industrial Injuries Advisory Council (1990) *Periodic Report*. London: HMSO.
3. Occupational Health Services (1978) *The way ahead*. London: HMSO.
4. Meredith SK, Taylor VM, McDonald JC (1991) Occupational respiratory disease in the United Kingdom 1989: a report to the British Thoracic Society and the Society of Occupational Medicine by the SWORD project group. *British Journal of Industrial Medicine*, **48**, 292.
5. Health and Safety Commission (1990) *Annual Report 1988–89*. London: HMSO.

6. Doll R, Peto R (1981) *The causes of cancer*. Oxford: Oxford University Press.
7. Wello M (1985) *Back pain*. Studies of current health problems, No 78. London: Office of Health Economics.
8. MacDonald EB, Dale JL (1984) Back pain: the risk factors and its prediction on work people. In *Occupational aspects of back disorders*. London: Society of Occupational Medicine.
9. Macbeth R (1952) Malignant disease of the para-nasal sinuses. *Journal of Laryngology*, **79**, 592.
10. Scott TS (1952) The incidence of bladder tumours in a dyestuff factory. *British Journal of Industrial Medicine*, **9**, 127.
11. Seaton A (1983) Coal and the lung. *Thorax*, **38**, 241.
12. British Coal Corporation Medical Service (1990) *Annual Report 1988–89*. London: British Coal Corporation.
13. Atherley G (1989) Prevention of occupational deafness: a coming crisis. *Journal of Occupational Medicine*, **31**(2), 139.
14. Fielding JE (1990) Worksite health promotion programs in the United States: progress, lessons and challenges. *Health Promotion International*, **5**(1), 75.

Further reading

Waldren HA (ed) (1989) *Occupational health practice* (3rd edn). London: Butterworths.
Swanson G (1988) Cancer prevention in the workplace and natural environment. *Cancer*, **62**, 1725.
World Health Organisation (1986). *Early detection of occupational diseases*. Geneva: WHO.
Faculty of Occupational Medicine (1988). *Fitness for work: the medical aspects*. Joint report of the Royal College of Physicians and the Faculty of Occupational Health (FC Edwards and RL McCallum, eds). Oxford: Oxford University Press.

Chapter 10: **Childhood**

1. Royal College of Physicians (1989) *Prenatal diagnosis and genetic screening: community and service implications*. A report of a working party. London: Royal College of Physicians of London.
2. Editorial (1990) Poverty and health in the 1990s. *British Medical Journal*, **301**, 349.
3. Whitehead M (1988) The health divide. In *Inequalities in health* (incorporating the Black Report). London: Penguin Books.
4. Butler J (1989) *Child health surveillance in primary care*. London: HMSO.
5. Pharoah POD (1986) Perspectives and patterns. *British Medical Bulletin*, **42**, 119.
6. Butler NR, Bonham DG (1963) *Perinatal mortality*. The first report of 1958 British Perinatal Mortality Survey. Edinburgh: Churchill Livingstone.

7. Chamberlain G, Philipp E, Howlett B, Masters K (1978) *British births 1970*. Vol 2: Obstetric care. London: Heinemann.
8. Hall DMB (1989) Birth asphyxia and cerebral palsy. *British Medical Journal*, **299**, 279.
9. Notzon FC, Placer PJ, Taffel SM (1987) Comparison of national caesarian rates. *New England Journal of Medicine*, **316**, 386.
10. Rosenblatt DB, Renshaw ME, Notarianni LT (1980) Pain relief in childbirth and its consequences for the infant. *Trends in Pharmacological Sciences*, September, 365.
11. Pharoah POD, Cooke T, Cooke RWI, Rosenbloom L (1990) Birthweight specific trends in cerebral palsy. *Archives of Disease in Childhood*, **65**, 602.
12. Klaus MN, Kennell JH (1976) *Maternal-infant bonding*. St Louis: CV Mosby.
13. Davies PA, Milner AD, Silverman D, Simpson H (1990) Monitoring and sudden infant death syndrome: an update. *Archives of Disease in Childhood*, **65**, 238.
14. Reznik VM, Murphy JL, Mendoza SA *et al* (1989) Following up of infants with obstructive uropathy detected *in utero* and treated surgically post-natally. *Journal of Paediatric Surgery*, **24**, 1289.
15. Editorial (1990) Antenatal screening for toxoplasmosis in the United Kingdom. *Lancet*, **ii**, 346.
16. Editorial (1989) Screening for congenital CMV. *Lancet*, **ii**, 599.
17. Royal College of Obstetricians and Gynaecologists (1990) *HIV infection in maternity care in gynaecology*. Revised report of the RCOG sub-committee on problems associated with AIDS in relation to obstetrics and gynaecology. London: Royal College of Obstetricians and Gynaecologists.
18. Taylor B, Wadsworth J (1987) Maternal smoking during pregnancy and lower respiratory tract illness in early life. *Archives of Disease in Childhood*, **62**, 786.
19. Taylor B, Wadsworth J, Golding J, Butler N (1982) Breastfeeding, bronchitis, and admissions for lower-respiratory illness and gastroenteritis during the first five years. *Lancet*, **i**, 1227.
20. Taylor B, Wadsworth J (1984) Breast feeding and child development at five years. *Developmental Medicine and Child Neurology*, **26**, 73.
21. Barker DJP, Winter PD, Osmond C *et al* (1989) Weight in infancy and death from ischaemic heart disease. *Lancet*, **ii**, 577.
22. Fergusson DM, Horwood LJ, Beautrais A (1981) Eczema and infant diet. *Clinical Allergy*, **11**, 325.
23. Chandra RK, Puri S, Hamed A (1989) Influence of maternal diet during lactation and use of formula feeds on development in atopic eczema in high risk infants. *British Medical Journal*, **299**, 228.
24. Wilson JM, Junger G (1968) *Principles and practice of screening for disease*. Public Health Papers. Geneva: WHO.
25. Leck I (1986) An epidemiological assessment of neonatal screening for dislocation of the hip. *Journal of the Royal College of Physicians*, **20**, 56.
26. Hall DMB (ed) (1989) *Health for all children: a programme for child health surveillance*. Oxford: Oxford University Press.
27. Puckering C (1989) Maternal depression. *Journal of Child Psychology and Psychiatry*, **30**, 807.
28. Thomson GO *et al* (1989) The Edinburgh lead study. *Journal of Child Psychology and Psychiatry*, **4**, 515.

29. Bewley B (1986) The epidemiology of adolescent behaviour problems. *British Medical Journal*, **42**, 200.
30. Charlton A (1988) Why do children smoke? In *Should prevention of coronary artery disease begin in childhood?* pp 21–27. Coronary Prevention Group.
31. Golding J (1986) Child health and the environment. *British Medical Bulletin*, **42**, 204.
32. Peckham C, Stark O, Moynihan D (1985) Obesity in school children: is there a case for screening? *Public Health*, **99**, 3.

Chapter 11: **Old age**

1. Grimley Evans J (1988) Ageing and disease. In *Research and the ageing population*. Ciba Foundation Symposium 134, pp 38–47. Chichester: Wiley-Liss.
2. Fairweather DS, Grimley Evans J (1990) Ageing. In *The metabolic and molecular basis of acquired disease* (eds RD Cohen, B Lewis, KGGM Alberti, AM Denman) pp 213–36. London: Bailliere Tindall.
3. Branch LG, Jette AM (1984) Personal health practices and mortality among the elderly. *American Journal of Public Health*, **74**, 1126.
4. Acland M (1854) *Memoir on the cholera at Oxford in the year 1854*. Oxford.
5. Fries JF (1980) Aging, natural death and the compression of morbidity. *New England Journal of Medicine*, **303**, 130.
6. Schneider EL, Brody JA (1983) Aging, natural death and the compression of morbidity: another view. *New England Journal of Medicine*, **309**, 854.
7. Katz S, Branch LG, Branson MH *et al* (1983) Active life expectancy. *New England Journal of Medicine*, **309**, 1218.
8. Staessen J, Fagard R, van Hoof R, Amery A (1988) Mortality in various intervention trials in elderly hypertensive patients: a review. *European Heart Journal*, **9**, 215.
9. SHEP (Systolic Hypertension in the Elderly Program) Cooperative Research Group (1991) Prevention of stroke by antihypertensive drug treatment in older persons with isolated systolic hypertension. Final results of SHEP. *Journal of the American Medical Association*, **165**, 3255.
10. Peto R. Personal Communication.
11. Hermanson B, Omenn GS, Kronmal RA *et al* (1988) Beneficial six-year outcome of smoking cessation in older men and women with coronary artery disease. Results from the CASS registry. *New England Journal of Medicine*, **319**, 1365.
12. Jajich CL, Ostfeld AM, Freeman DH (1984) Smoking and coronary heart disease mortality in the elderly. *Journal of the American Medical Association*, **252**, 2831.
13. Grimley Evans J, Prudham D, Wandless I (1980) Risk factors for stroke in the elderly. In: *The ageing brain: neurological and mental disturbances* (eds G Barbagallo-Sangiorgi, AN Exton-Smith), pp 113–25. New York: Plenum Press.
14. Petersen P, Madsen EB, Brun B *et al* (1987) Silent cerebral infarction in chronic atrial fibrillation. *Stroke*, **18**, 1098.
15. Wolf PA, Kannel WB, McGee DL *et al* (1983) Duration of atrial fibrillation and imminence of stroke: the Framingham study. *Stroke*, **14**, 664.

16. Gjaweski J, Singer R (1981) Mortality in an insured population with atrial fibrillation. *Journal of the American Medical Association*, **245**, 1540.
17. The Boston Area Anticoagulation Trial for Atrial Fibrillation Investigators (1990) The effect of low-dose warfarin on the risk of stroke in patients with non-rheumatic atrial fibrillation. *New England Journal of Medicine*, **323**, 1505.
18. Wickramasinghe LSP, Basu SK, Bansal SK (1988) Long-term anticoagulant therapy in elderly patients. *Age and Ageing*, **17**, 388.
19. Winner SJ, Morgan CA, Grimley Evans J (1989) Perimenopausal risk of falling and incidence of distal forearm fracture. *British Medical Journal*, **298**, 1486.
20. Grimley Evans J (1990) The significance of osteoporosis. In *Osteoporosis 1990* (ed R Smith), pp 1–8. London: Royal College of Physicians.
21. Radebaugh TS, Hadley E, Suzman R (eds) (1985) Falls in the elderly: biologic and behavioural aspects. *Clinics in Geriatric Medicine*, **1**, 3.
22. Gray JAM, Bassey EJ, Young A (1985) The risks of inactivity. In *Prevention of disease in the elderly* (ed. JAM Gray), pp 78–94. Edinburgh: Churchill Livingstone.
23. Council of Scientific Affairs, American Medical Association (1983) Medical evaluations of healthy persons. *Journal of the American Medical Association*, **249**, 1626.
24. House JS, Landis KR, Umberson D (1988) Social relationships and health. *Science*, **241**, 540.
25. Bastow MD, Rawlings J, Allison SP (1983) Undernutrition, hypothermia, and injury in elderly women with fractured femur: and injury response to altered metabolism? *Lancet*, **1**, 143.
26. COMA (In press). *The nutrition of the elderly*. A report of the Committee on Medical Aspects of Food Policy. London: Department of Health.
27. Krall EA, Sahyoun N, Tannenbaum S *et al* (1989) Effect of vitamin D intake on seasonal variation in parathyroid hormone secretion in post-menopausal women. *New England Journal of Medicine*, **321**, 1777.
28. Kane R, Kane R (1986) Self-care and health care: inseparable but equal for the well-being of the old. In *Self-care and health in old age* (eds K Dean, T Hickey, BE Holstein), pp 251–83. London: Croom Helm.
29. Shanas E, Townsend P, Wedderburn D *et al* (1968) *Old people in three industrial societies*. London: Routledge and Kegan Paul.

RCP paperbacks
